Th

# Pilates
Prescription for
# Back Pain

# The
# **Pilates**
# Prescription for
# **Back Pain**

*A Comprehensive Program for*

*Developing and Maintaining a Healthy Back*

*Lynne Robinson, Helge Fisher, Paul Massey*

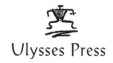

Ulysses Press

Published in the United States by
Ulysses Press
P.O. Box 3440
Berkeley, CA 94703
www.ulyssespress.com

First published in the United Kingdom in 2002 by Pan Books
an imprint of Pan Macmillan Ltd.

Library of Congress Card Number 2003109421
ISBN 1-56975-394-6

Printed in Canada by Transcontinental Printing

10 9 8 7 6 5 4 3 2 1

U.S. Editorial and Production: Steven Schwartz, Lily Chou, Lisa Kester, Laura Brancella

Distributed in the United States by Publishers Group West
and in Canada by Raincoast Books

Please Note
This book has been written and published strictly for informational purposes, and in no
way should be used as a substitute for consultation with health care professionals. You
should not consider educational material herein to be the practice of medicine or to
replace consultation with a physician or other medical practitioner. The author and
publisher are providing you with information in this work so that you can have the
knowledge and can choose, at your own risk, to act on that knowledge. The author and
publisher also urge all readers to be aware of their health status and to consult health
care professionals before beginning any health program.

# Contents

# Acknowledgements

I was in my early thirties when I first began to suffer with back pain. Years of appalling posture, lack of exercise, two large babies, and two abdominal operations had taken their toll on my body. The final straw was an afternoon on the golf driving range when I managed to herniate a disc! I tried various therapists and practitioners but the pain kept recurring after treatment. It was while we were living in Sydney, Australia, that my osteopath Philip Latey recommended I try Pilates. I had never heard of it but I was desperate to do something to help myself rather than rely on therapists to "fix" me each time. Within twenty minutes of the first class with Penny Latey I knew this was right for me, and so began my new life . . . .

This, then, is the perfect opportunity to thank all the practitioners who have worked on me and who have worked with me. Philip Latey, Piers Chandler, Jacqueline Knox and Paul Massey have been endlessly generous with both their knowledge and support. Gordon Thomson was brave enough to take me on when we returned to the U.K. He has been a source of inspiration and a wonderful friend. I must also thank my co-author Helge Fisher for sharing her expert knowledge with us. Everyone needs to practice regularly and it helps to have correction and guidance, and this is where Lisa Bradshaw and the staff at our South Kensington studio have been amazingly patient and understanding with me (and my body). Finally, I want to mention all the Body Control Pilates teachers who are doing such a fantastic job helping people overcome back pain all over the world. Thank you! You are the real stars!

**Lynne Robinson**

I would like to thank my many patients from whom I learn so much and without whom this book would not have been possible. For the support of SD, my family and friends, whose inspiration and advice are always welcome and thought about when given.

To the staff and colleagues at Body Control Pilates, who keep the ball rolling to improve the application of Pilates, and the team at the Partnership, Ashford, for sharing their clinical experience in back-care management.

Thanks to the publishers, Macmillan, for all their help and encouragement.

**Paul Massey**

There are many people who taught me to follow my heart and believe in a vision and I would like to thank them all.

Listening to my heart is not always easy and I am full of gratitude towards my children Naomi and Amina and my husband Paul, who are patient and understanding when I am struggling.

I would also like to thank the teachers who inspire me: Eric Franklin, Kelly Kane, Sasha, Paul McLinden and Anja Saunders, and my support team Andrea, Iren and Lynda.

**Helge Fisher**

A big thank you from all of us to Moira Rees MCSP SRP (Reform: Physiotherapy and Pilates Studio, Bishops Waltham) for reading the manuscript and giving her highly valued opinion.

# Introduction

The chances are that if you have picked up or bought this book you are suffering from, or know someone who is suffering from, back pain. You are not alone! Most of us will experience back trouble at some point in our lives. Statistics related to back pain tell their own story: surveys show that in the United States nearly 50 percent of adults have, in any given year, back pain lasting more than one day – that's about 97 million people! In half of these cases, the pain lasted more than four weeks. Back pain is no indication of age, sex, social group, profession or level of fitness – men and women are equally likely to suffer and, while it is those in the age range 45–64 who suffer most frequently, one third of adults aged under twenty-five also claim to have regular back pain in spite of the fact that there has been excellent medical research into the causes of back pain (see references on page 227) and that state-of-the-art diagnostic equipment has never been more accessible.

Despite these advances, over one million people are disabled by back pain at some time in their lives and, in economic terms, the cost to the nation of back problems is estimated to be between $20 to $50 billion per annum, the vast majority of which is due to absence from work. Back pain is second only to the common cold as one of the major reasons why we miss work. Mind-boggling figures indeed. The bottom line is that although we may now be better than ever at diagnosing and understanding why we have back pain, most of us are still not taking the right steps either to prevent back problems in the first place or to prevent their recurrence.

At the end of the day, this is the responsibility of the back-pain sufferer him- or herself. A doctor, physiotherapist, osteopath or chiropractor may be able to treat you with medication, massage, manipulation, traction, heat, acupuncture and more, but no one can do your exercises for you, nor can they follow you around reminding you to sit up tall! It is time for us to take responsibility for our own bodies and this is precisely why we have written this book: to serve as a self-help manual for people with back problems or people who wish to prevent back trouble from starting. The advice here is not a substitute for proper medical diagnosis or treatment, but it can be used to help you understand why you have a problem, to help speed your recovery and to help prevent recurrence. Be warned, though, that it is not going to be easy. There is no quick fix – it will require you to devote time to exercising and to make some changes to your lifestyle. That's the bad news. The good news is that it can work for you, not only improving the way you feel and the way you move, but also the way you look.

A new back, a new body and perhaps even a completely new way of life is just a few pages away . . . .

# How the Back Works and Why It Sometimes Goes Wrong

*Joseph Pilates would say that "you are as old as your spine" and that "a healthy back means a healthy spine."*

## Get to Know Your Spine

In a healthy back there are three natural curves and groups of muscles that work to support these curves.

### The Vertebral Bodies

The curves of the spine may alter for various reasons, including, for example, poor posture or a change in muscle balance, and this can result in back problems. We will explore this later, but first let's take a closer look at the vertebrae themselves (see next page).

**Curves of the spine**

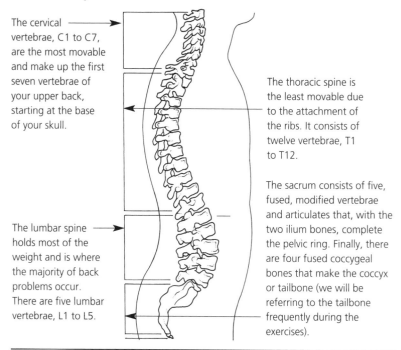

The cervical vertebrae, C1 to C7, are the most movable and make up the first seven vertebrae of your upper back, starting at the base of your skull.

The thoracic spine is the least movable due to the attachment of the ribs. It consists of twelve vertebrae, T1 to T12.

The lumbar spine holds most of the weight and is where the majority of back problems occur. There are five lumbar vertebrae, L1 to L5.

The sacrum consists of five, fused, modified vertebrae and articulates that, with the two ilium bones, complete the pelvic ring. Finally, there are four fused coccygeal bones that make the coccyx or tailbone (we will be referring to the tailbone frequently during the exercises).

These vertebral bodies can be compared to a child's building blocks stacked one on top of the other. The area behind the vertebral body consists of a ring of bone that circles around the spinal cord and has small projections of bone from each of the outside corners. The projections to the side are called the transverse processes and the projection from the back is called the spinous process. These are the bony knobs that can be felt in the back. The function of these bony projections is to act as points of attachment for muscles in order to allow for movement of the vertebrae and to help prevent them from locking together – they also prevent you from bending too far backward.

When the vertebrae are stacked on top of one another, the bony ring that lies behind the vertebral body creates a tube – the spinal canal – along which the spinal cord, consisting of a bundle of spinal nerves, runs to emerge at the level of the second lumbar vertebrae, where it hangs down like a horse's tail (cauda equina).

Filaments in parts of the spinal cord form the spinal nerve roots that leave the spinal canal from a notch behind the vertebral body on the level under the corresponding vertebra. So, for example, the root for the second lumbar nerve comes out under the second lumbar vertebra at the space at that level.

**The vertebral body**

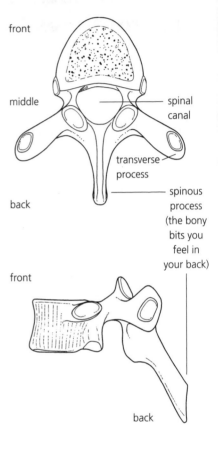

As we can only really feel and see the spinous processes of the spine, most of us believe the spine to be far back in the trunk. In reality, however, the twenty-four weight-bearing bodies of the vertebrae and the intervertebral discs are quite central in the body.

If you place your fingers into your navel, depending on your build, the main vertebral bodies are about two to four inches from your fingers.

# Spinal Discs

In between each vertebra lie the discs, cushions of elastic tissue that act as shock absorbers between each vertebra, protecting the spine from the impact on it as we walk, run, jump and fall, and permitting, normally, movement in every direction.

Each disc has three components:

- the annulus fibrosis
- the nucleus pulposus
- the vertebral end plates

The outer rim casing of the spinal disc is called the annulus fibrosis. The annulus consists of layers of fibrous tissue arranged in concentric bands acting like a corset and holding the nucleus in place. When the spine has to bear weight, the nucleus of the disc spreads out and the annulus bulges, acting like a hydraulic sack by dispersing the pressure of the weight from the body above.

The central area of the disc is called the nucleus pulposus and consists of a hydrophilic (water-attracting) substance that enables the nucleus to alter its water-retaining capacity depending on the physical force placed on the whole disc. So an increase in pressure results in a loss of fluid. Certain positions such as sitting, or movements such as bending forward, exert extra pressure on the discs (see the chart below).

Did you know that you are about half an inch taller in the mornings than in the evenings? This is simply because you lose fluid in the discs during the day (unless you spend it lying down!). When you lie down, the fluid is absorbed back into the discs. The amount of fluid and therefore the load-bearing capacity of the discs is also reduced with age, which makes us more vulnerable to injury as we grow older.

The final part of the disc is the vertebral end plates, which are formed of hyaline cartilage on the surface of the vertebrae. Parts of them act to facilitate the exchange of fluid between the bony vertebral body and the disc. They also protect the vertebral body from excessive pressure.

Let's take a closer look at how different positions and movements can affect the disc. It is easy to see how sitting all day, especially in a slouched position, is going to put pressure on the discs. It is far better to vary position frequently.

See next page.

**Side view of a vertebra and disc**

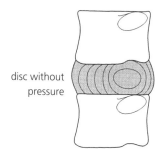

disc without pressure

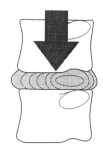

when pressure is applied the disc bulges

## How different postures affect disc pressure

(Adapted from A. Nachemson, "The Lumbar Spine in Orthopaedic Challenge," 1976, *Spine*, 1, 59–71.)

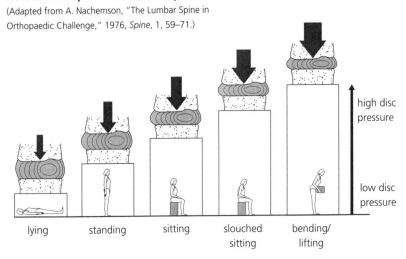

| lying | standing | sitting | slouched sitting | bending/ lifting |

high disc pressure

low disc pressure

As we get older, most of us will suffer from general wear and tear of the discs. Although minor disc problems are common, few of us heed the initial warning signs, for example, increasing backache, strain in the back following awkward movement, painful tension in the butt or cramp-like symptoms in the leg. The majority of problems seem to occur in the most flexible parts of our back such as the lower back or the neck.

A fairly common condition is the one known as a "slipped disc." This is a misleading term, however, and does not accurately describe what happens; the proper name is "prolapsed disc" and it is a condition that can cause severe back problems. Essentially, due to excessive pressure (quite often bending forward and rotating – see above) the outer casing of the disc splits and the nucleus protrudes and can press against a nerve root. This is very painful and needs proper medical diagnosis. Of course, there are less severe disc problems, such as bulging discs.

**Healthy disc**

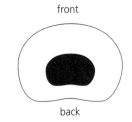

front

back

**Unhealthy disc**

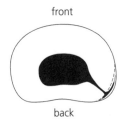

front

back

when a disc bulges, the nucleus travels down a tear in the annulus part of the disc

# Facet Joints

The facet joints are the small joints at the back of the spine where bone meets bone from the neighboring vertebrae. They are coated with slippery cartilage and lubricated by synovial fluid, both of which help them slide easily on each other. The facet joints form a chain up the spine so the joint surfaces link together. They act to prevent you from overstretching your discs by bending too far backward or twisting around too far. When you bend forward, the facet joints open and allow more rotation (see below). If you have good spinal alignment, then the facet joints do not have to bear too much weight.

There are several reasons why you may develop facet-joint problems. If you have an excessive lordosis in the lumbar spine (an increased hollow in the low back) then the facet joints may have more weight to bear and, since they are not designed to do this, problems may result. Too much or uneven pressure through poor posture is therefore the most common cause of facet-joint problems; the joint becomes inflamed and you may feel a deep ache or pain over the joint or you may feel referred pain (see page 41). Other common causes of facet-joint problems include disc shrinkage and muscle imbalance.

**Side view of the spine**

**Back view of the spine**

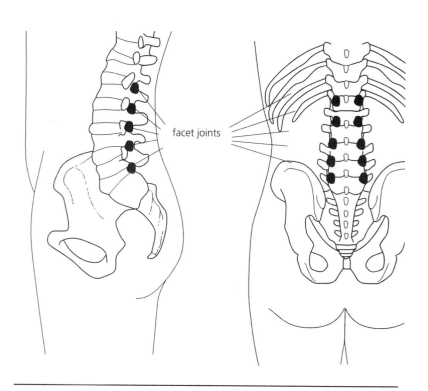

facet joints

## Spinal Ligaments

Spinal ligaments are cords of fibrous tissue running the length of the spine and keeping the spinal segments together. The anterior longitudinal ligament is attached to the front of the vertebral bodies and acts as a brake when you extend your back (bend backward). The posterior longitudinal ligament, which is attached to the back of the vertebral bodies, and the supraspinous ligament run along the tips of the spinous processes and act as a brake when you bend forward. In addition to controlling movement, the ligaments also provide sensory feedback to help determine where you are in space (proprioception).

The role of the ligaments is to keep the individual segments of the spine together, so that when they are stretched or shortened there will be a change in mobility. Ligament stress can result if these cords are stretched or shortened too far, usually due to poor posture. Stretched ligaments can lead to hypermobility (too much movement), tight ligaments can lead to hypomobility (too little movement).

**The spinal ligaments**

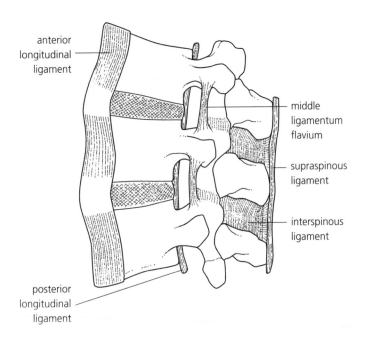

anterior longitudinal ligament

middle ligamentum flavium

supraspinous ligament

interspinous ligament

posterior longitudinal ligament

# Spinal Nerves

Through the center of the spine lies the spinal canal, and through this runs the spinal cord, a collection of nerves whose job it is to carry messages to and from the brain coordinating muscle action and sensory signals and relaying sensations such as touch, pain and temperature. Two nerves emerge from the spinal cord at the level of each vertebra via an exit point called the intervertebral foramina, which is bordered on one side by the facet joint and on the other by the disc. One nerve exits to the right and one to the left, each going to a specific area of the body.

If a nerve becomes trapped at the exit point then pain may be referred to the leg along the sciatic nerve – this is commonly called sciatica.

**Causes of sciatic pain**

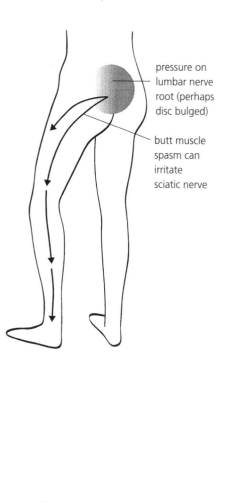

pressure on lumbar nerve root (perhaps disc bulged)

butt muscle spasm can irritate sciatic nerve

**The sciatic nerve**

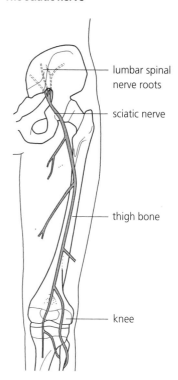

lumbar spinal nerve roots

sciatic nerve

thigh bone

knee

# Scoliosis

Scoliosis is a curvature of the spine with a lateral curve one way and a rotation the other. C-shape spines are often referred to as scoliosis, but they are in fact "lists."

Scoliosis often develops in childhood and can lead to structural problems of the pelvis, vertebra and thoracic cage. Scoliosis can be the result of injury: we tend to avoid the full use of that part or side of the back which is painful – resulting compensatory posture leads to scoliosis.

The very nature of scoliosis is such that a general prescription is meaningless because every individual's curve differs and requires specialist diagnosis. However, the overall lengthening, stability and breathing exercise contained in this program could be beneficial.

**C-shape and S-shape scoliosis**

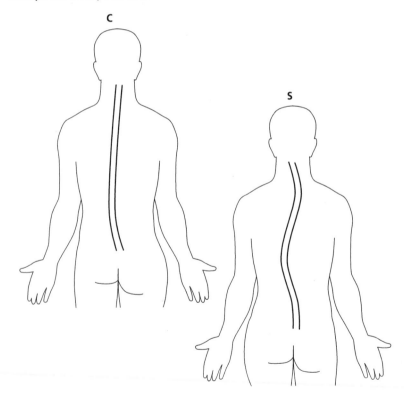

# Sacroiliac Joints

The sacroiliac joints (si joints) are the link between the pelvis and the spine. Usually these joints are very strong and there is not much movement in them. Sometimes we can strain the ligaments in the joints by twisting or falling, for example, stepping or slipping awkwardly off the curb. Problems can occur quite often throughout and after pregnancy, when hormonal changes during pregnancy cause the ligaments to soften, making the pelvic girdle particularly at risk. Strong core muscles, such as the transversus abdominis muscles, strengthened by Pilates exercises, can play a vital role in avoiding these problems.

**The sacroiliac joints**

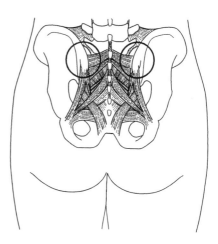

## Osteoarthritis

Sadly this condition is unavoidable to a degree. It is a term used to describe degenerative damage to bone and cartilage and is simply a part of growing older. Its onset can be delayed by keeping flexible, strong and mobile. Many of our Body Control Pilates exercises work on the mobility of the joints, especially the spine, which helps to keep them well lubricated. Furthermore, correct alignment of the joints, especially working in neutral, which will be explained later, will help reduce wear and tear because the bones will sit comfortably together with less stress. Finally, by strengthening the muscles around the joints themselves, you can help prevent further degeneration. If you have osteoarthritis we recommend that you avoid any exercises using weights.

## Osteoporosis

About 30 percent of women and 5 percent of men will suffer in later life from osteoporosis or brittle bone disease, which is defined as a loss of bone mineral resulting in thinning of the bone. Although bone looks very solid it is in fact full of holes rather like coral; any thinning of this sort of structure is therefore very dangerous.

**Healthy bone**

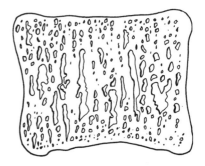

**Brittle bone**

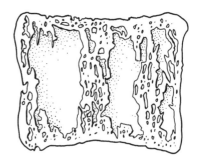

Bone health is maintained by good nutrition, which provides an adequate supply of minerals and vitamins, especially vitamin D; by the proper amounts of several hormones; and by the amount of stress the bone is put under. This is one type of stress that is good for us! Bones become thicker and stronger when they are stressed because stress produces electrical effects in the bone that, in turn, encourage bone growth. If there is no stress, the bone will be less dense and weaker.

During our lives there is a constant turnover of bone. Up until the age of thirty-five we lose as much old bone each year as we make new bone, so there is no problem. From then on, however, we tend to lose about 1 percent of our bone mass each year until women reach menopause, when bone loss accelerates with a typical further loss of 2 percent per year for up to ten years. By the age of seventy approximately one third of bone mass will be lost – no wonder granny appears to be shrinking!

We have two types of bone, trabecular (accounting for 20 percent of our bone mass) and cortical (80 percent). Trabecular bone is found mainly in the spine, pelvis and at the ends of long bones such as the head of the thigh bone, which is the bone that suffers most from a loss of density after menopause. Cortical bone is found in the shafts of the long bones and in the skull, and here bone loss is more gradual.

Most fractures that occur through osteoporosis are at the wrist, the spine and the hip.

Bone mass is affected by:

- Hormonal status – menopausal women in particular suffer from bone loss, which accelerates with the decline in the ovarian hormone, estrogen.

- Dietary intake – especially the inclusion of naturally occurring plant estrogens and calcium in our diet during our growing years.

- Genetic factors – which determine the size of our bones and muscles.

- Physical activity – particularly weight-bearing exercise.

Recent research has shown that regular weight-bearing exercise can help prevent the onset of osteoporosis. The earlier we start gentle weight training the better; it is not too early even in our teens because we are then laying good foundations for the future.

Many of the exercises we describe involve the use of light hand and leg weights and are perfect for the prevention of brittle bones. If you already have osteoporosis, you will need to consult your medical practitioner since the exercises may not be suitable for your condition.

As a general rule, it is wise to avoid all exercises that involve flexing the body (bending forward) because this will further encourage the hunched over posture associated with osteoporosis. So avoid Curl Ups and any exercises that involve lifting the head from the floor, as well as Roll Downs. In place of these, because you want to promote lengthening in the spine and correct its forward rounding, a gentle extension of the back is indicated, using, for example, the Diamond Press and the Dart.

# The Movements of the Spine

Now that you know what the spine consists of, you need to understand the effect that different movements have on it. Basically, you can flex or bend forward, extend or bend backward, rotate or twist and laterally flex or side bend.

**Flexion (forward bending)**

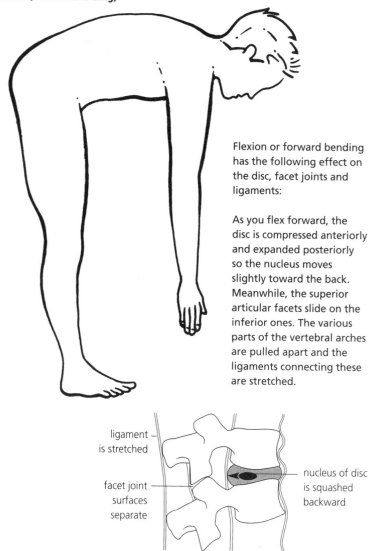

Flexion or forward bending has the following effect on the disc, facet joints and ligaments:

As you flex forward, the disc is compressed anteriorly and expanded posteriorly so the nucleus moves slightly toward the back. Meanwhile, the superior articular facets slide on the inferior ones. The various parts of the vertebral arches are pulled apart and the ligaments connecting these are stretched.

ligament is stretched

facet joint surfaces separate

nucleus of disc is squashed backward

**Extension (backward bending)**

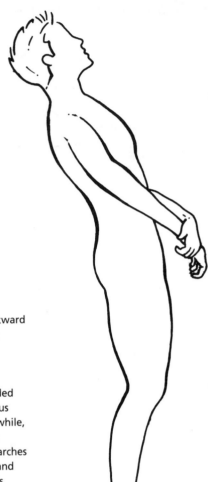

With extension or backward bending the following happens:

The disc is compressed posteriorly and expanded anteriorly so the nucleus moves forward. Meanwhile, the articular facets are pressed together, the arches move closer together and the posterior ligaments are relaxed. The anterior longitudinal ligament is stretched.

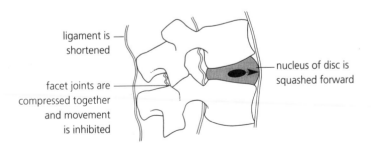

ligament is shortened

facet joints are compressed together and movement is inhibited

nucleus of disc is squashed forward

## Lateral flexion (side bend)

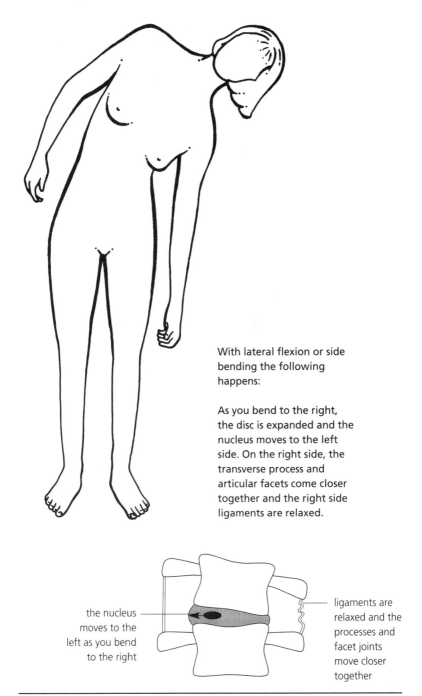

With lateral flexion or side bending the following happens:

As you bend to the right, the disc is expanded and the nucleus moves to the left side. On the right side, the transverse process and articular facets come closer together and the right side ligaments are relaxed.

the nucleus moves to the left as you bend to the right

ligaments are relaxed and the processes and facet joints move closer together

## Rotation

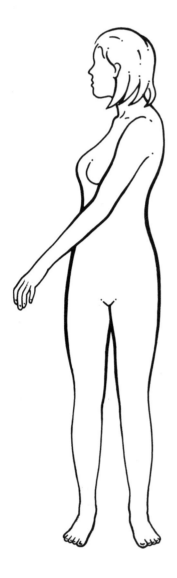

When you rotate the spine, you stretch and twist the fibers of the disc and there is an overall reduction in the height of the disc, resulting in some compression of the nucleus. Meanwhile, the transverse and spinous processes are moved apart and their connecting ligaments are stretched.

Having studied how different movements affect the nucleus of the disc, you can see why certain combined movements such as forward bending and twisting can be potentially harmful. Remember this next time you bend down to lift your two-year-old out of the stroller and put her into the car seat. It is not usually a single action that causes the damage, but the accumulative effect of repeatedly bending, twisting and lifting.

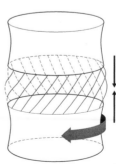

pressure on the disc results in compression of the nucleus. The processes are moved apart by rotation and the ligaments are stretched

# The Muscles and Sound Movement Patterns

Of course, none of the above movements take place without the involvement of the muscles that work together in groups to move our bones. They work as a team. With everything working correctly and firing up in the right order or sequence you have a good pattern of use, or sound recruitment pattern, and normal movement. That's exactly how we used to move as children. In the next chapter we will be looking at how and why normal movement is lost, but, for now, we should investigate the three components to normal movement.

- The Control System:
  the nervous system

- The Active System:
  muscle recruitment

- The Passive System:
  the skeletal frame ligaments

For normal movement to exist, you need these three systems to be functioning efficiently with no injuries or problems. If any one part is not working properly, then problems arise.

Movement depends on the constant flow of messages to and from the brain via the nervous system: input and output. The brain remembers patterns of movement rather than individual contractions and these become locked in the memory banks and are performed habitually. If the brain receives the right messages we move well. But similarly the brain also remembers and stores bad patterns of movement! This is why good body use and improved body awareness are so important. More about that later!

**Transversus abdominis, your natural girdle of strength**

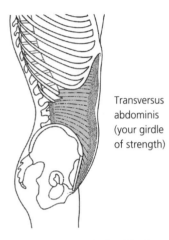

Transversus
abdominis
(your girdle
of strength)

Multifidus.
As you zip up
and hollow (see
page 49),
multifidus
is engaged,
stabilizing your
lumbar spine

For the spine to be healthy it must be in a balanced state where both the spine itself and its nerves are protected from compression by abnormal stress, permitting it to move freely without problems.

The spine itself is completely surrounded by muscles, to the front, back and sides. These muscles have a dual role:

- To keep the spine stable by giving it support so that the limbs can move efficiently – these are referred to as stabilizing or fixating muscles.

- To move the spine in different directions – referred to as mobilizing muscles

The importance of the deep stabilizing muscles is becoming increasingly clear in medical research. Let's say you want to reach up to take a book from a high shelf. Which muscles do you think would be the first to engage? The hand or shoulder muscles perhaps? The answer is the deep postural muscles – in other words, those supporting the spine.

Think about it – it makes sense – you don't want to fall over while you reach up. These deep muscles – the transversus abdominis, the pelvic floor muscles and a deep back muscle called multifidus – are the ones that stabilize the lumbar spine, ensuring that one vertebra doesn't shear too far off its neighbor. These muscles engage to form a natural corset, a "girdle of strength," around your center so that the movement can take place easily, smoothly and safely. You must have this stable base in the same way that a tower crane needs a stable base while the long arm moves around.

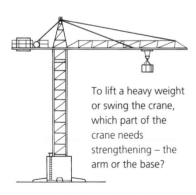

To lift a heavy weight or swing the crane, which part of the crane needs strengthening – the arm or the base?

Problems can arise when these deep stabilizing muscles are not working correctly. This can happen for a variety of reasons, but it is usually when your body is held out of its correct alignment in incorrect positions for sustained periods of time (see figure on next page). The stabilizing muscles are held on a stretch and are therefore weakened. Other muscles are then "forced" to take over the stabilizing role and the wrong muscles start doing the wrong job. We then have the birth of a faulty muscle recruitment pattern: a pattern of misuse.

In an ideal world muscles designed to stabilize will stabilize, those designed to mobilize will mobilize. Returning to our image of the crane, the stabilizers are the stable base, the mobilizers make the large sweeping movements of the arm of the crane. Some muscles work as stabilizers in some movements and mobilizers in others. If, however, a deep stabilizing muscle is not functioning properly, a mobilizer may take on a stabilizing role, changing its fiber types and no longer able to work efficiently as a mobilizer. For example, if the muscles that stabilize your spine (transversus and multifidus) are not working correctly, the more superficial mobilizing muscles – the erector spinae, which is the superficial muscle at the side of your spine – will take on a stabilizing role and, as a result, become tighter. No wonder your low back always feels tight! And remember, this type of imbalance may occur anywhere in the body where stabilizing and mobilizing muscles are not performing efficiently.

The two types of muscles have different characteristics. Stabilizing muscles have to work for long periods of time, they have to hold tone and need endurance, they usually lie deeper within the body, and are often shorter in length than mobilizing muscles. They work at about 20 to 30 percent of their full efficiency (Maximum Voluntary Contraction – MVC) and have a predominance of slow twitch fibers. These enable the muscle to contract slowly in order to sustain a continuous endurance. A steady flow of oxygen is needed to help maintain this process.

Mobilizing muscles, on the other hand, make big movements, such as moving the limbs around. In order to make these movements they work in phases, turning on and off. They tend to be more superficial, lie closer to the surface of the body than the stabilizing muscles, and are usually quite long. They fatigue quickly and work at between 40 to 100 percent of their full efficiency – MVC – and have a predominance of fast twitch fibers.

A very common muscle imbalance that most of us can identify with is tight hamstrings. Hamstring muscles, which for many movements act as mobilizing muscles enabling large movements, are often "obliged" to take on the role of stabilizing the pelvis because the deep gluteals (butt) are too weak. Consequently, the hamstrings tighten and shorten. No amount of stretching will lengthen them while they have to keep stabilizing. The solution to this problem would be to strengthen the deep gluteals and then the hamstrings can let go.

When stabilizing and mobilizing muscles work perfectly at their own jobs, the body is balanced: all the groups of muscles work in synergy and joints are held in their most favorable position, which is their natural "neutral" position.

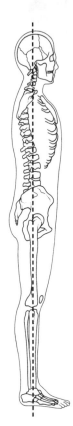

Figure one
Ideal plumb line alignment

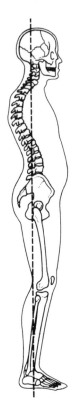

Figure two
Kyphosis-Lordosis

You can see this in a person with perfect posture. By studying the figure in the diagram, you can see that all the joints in the body are held in their optimum natural position. When this person moves, with good muscle recruitment and with the stabilizing muscles working correctly, there is going to be minimal wear and tear on the joints. Good input is received by the brain and locked into the memory banks.

Compare this picture with the one of the person above. Here, most of the joints are held out of their natural neutral positions because of existing muscle imbalances. Those all-important stabilizing muscles are held on a stretch and thus weakened. Tight, shortened muscles and weak, lengthened muscles, inefficient stabilizers and overactive mobilizers equate with faulty recruitment patterns that feel like normal movement. These patterns of misuse are repeated and provide "input" into the nervous system, which accepts them as "normal"; the brain thus receives bad input that it then locks into its memory bank.

The beauty of the Body Control Pilates method is that the exercises work by building strength from the inside out – not just in the trunk, but in the whole body. Not only are you taught how to position your body correctly in good postural alignment, you are also taught how to engage and strengthen those all-important stabilizing muscles.

The ultimate goal of Body Control Pilates exercises is to restore natural, normal movement patterns to the body.

**Pilates exercises work on strengthening these stabilizing muscles**

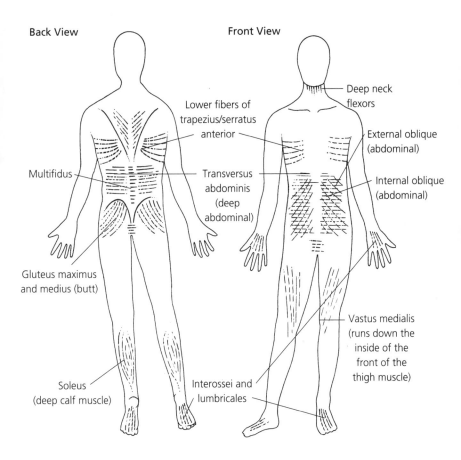

Back View

Front View

Lower fibers of trapezius/serratus anterior

Deep neck flexors

External oblique (abdominal)

Multifidus

Transversus abdominis (deep abdominal)

Internal oblique (abdominal)

Gluteus maximus and medius (butt)

Vastus medialis (runs down the inside of the front of the thigh muscle)

Soleus (deep calf muscle)

Interossei and lumbricales

# Why Do So Many People Get Back Pain?

As practitioners working with back-pain sufferers, believe us, we get some very strange explanations as to why and how our clients' back pains started! The most common usually includes the phrase, "I was just bending down. . . ." Perhaps the most bizarre was, "I was standing there peeling potatoes and I felt my back go. . . ."

In this chapter, we investigate some of the reasons back problems occur. A lot of them develop over a period of time and finally a single occurrence is the last straw – the one that breaks the poor camel's back! We often choose not to notice the small warning signs and therefore blame a particular activity or specific movement that seems to have caused the crisis. But, actually, it is that one movement which has made us stop and acknowledge that something is wrong; the problem usually started much earlier.

There are many reasons why people get backache. But, broadly speaking, they can be divided into:

- new use
- misuse
- overuse
- abuse
- disuse

Let's take a look at each one.

## New Use

A common cause of backache is starting up a new activity, something that we may not have done before. Perhaps we have just moved house and have decided to decorate or clear the garden. Perhaps we have had a bout of conscience and joined the local gym, signing up for every class on the schedule! Frequently, we may not feel so much as a twinge at the time, but the next day . . . .

## Misuse

This is the cumulative effect of bad body use over a long period of time. It usually means that we have very poor body awareness and postural alignment. As a result, our movement patterns are faulty.

## Overuse

By this, we mean the repetitive use of one muscle group creating an imbalance in the body. There are numerous examples of this in all walks of life, from the supermarket checkout person repeatedly twisting at the register, the shoe salesman eternally bending down to fit shoes, to the professional golfer bending and rotating as he swings, the tennis player serving again and again – you get the picture.

## Abuse

Lifting a piano would be included in this category. We are all guilty at some point of pushing our bodies too far, of asking too much. It doesn't have to be a piano, it may be a dining table or a crate of beer. It isn't necessarily lifting, either, for we can just as easily strain by over-reaching, twisting or, worse still, combining all three. At the end of the book, there is a chapter explaining how to do these activities safely.

## Disuse

Lack of exercise in itself may not cause a back problem, but a problem may easily result when we attempt an activity requiring a certain degree of strength or flexibility that we have long since lost through lack of exercise.

The problem is often an amalgamation of all of the above, but we can also add the following contributory factors:

## ENVIRONMENTAL FACTORS

Our surroundings and furniture can have both a positive and a negative effect on our bodies. Our workstation, chair, car seat, couch, bed – if these are well-designed and we maintain good posture, we may avoid problems. But far too often this is not the case, or we have bought furniture for looks rather than comfort, and we accordingly spend far too long in sustained, held positions without free movement.

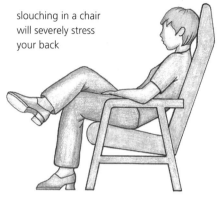

slouching in a chair will severely stress your back

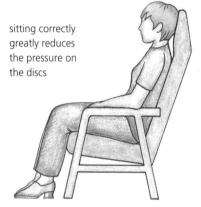

sitting correctly greatly reduces the pressure on the discs

## FASHION AND CULTURE

We are all victims here, knowingly too. Look at how high-heeled shoes alter the angle of the pelvis and spine. (For one wonderful season, though, backpacks were all the rage so we carried our belongings squarely on both shoulders rather than on one side. See next page.)

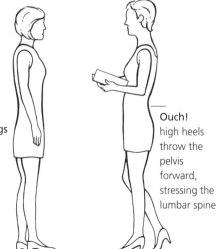

with heels at the right height, the pelvis and spine stay in good neutral alignment

Ouch! high heels throw the pelvis forward, stressing the lumbar spine

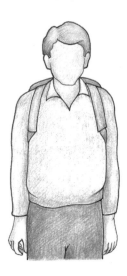
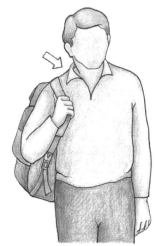

## EMOTIONAL STRESS

Whenever we are stressed we tend to tense our muscles. That's why we often suffer from tension headaches, because the whole angle of the head and neck is altered under stress, resulting in a build-up of tension at the back of the neck and around the jaw. We can also feel this tension in the upper shoulders. Anxiety really makes us "tighten up." This can easily build up over a period of time and contribute to muscle imbalances. This is why Relaxation is the first of the Eight Principles of the Pilates method!

All of the above can alter the way we are – changing our movement patterns and our posture and thus opening the door to potential back disorders.

Many of the problems seen by physiotherapists, chiropractors and osteopaths are related to poor posture. We looked briefly in the previous chapter at good postural alignment but now is the perfect time to look more closely at the different postural types and their muscle imbalances.

**Relaxed**

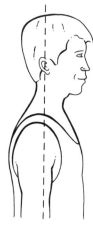

**Stressed**

we carry tension in the neck and shoulders when stressed

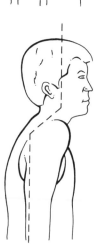

# *Ideal Posture*

With "ideal posture" the forces of gravity are evenly distributed through the body and all joints are in their neutral zone. There will be minimal wear and tear on these structures and the natural balance and correct length of the muscles is maintained. Because muscles are balanced, movement patterns are normal. All vital organs are properly placed and not constricted so they function better.

Notice the points of the body through which an imaginary plumb line (see page 20) falls:

- the ear lobe

- the bodies of the cervical vertebrae (the neck)

- the tip of the shoulder

- dividing the thorax (ribcage) in half

- the bodies of the lumbar vertebrae

- slightly behind the hip joint

- slightly in front of the center of the knee joint

- slightly in front of the outside ankle bone (lateral malleolus)

This, then, is what we should all aspire to, bearing in mind that we each have our own distinctive body shape, size and dimensions.

The head is in good neutral alignment, neither tilted forward or back.

The shoulder blades lie flat against the thorax.

The ribcage is not compressed so breathing is more efficient.

The spine retains its natural curves.

The pelvis is in its natural neutral position (the anterior superior iliac spine is in line with the pubis symphysis).

The knee joints are in a line and not hyperextended (locked back).

The lower leg is vertical and at a right angle to the sole of the foot.

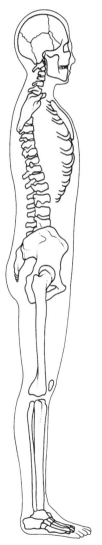

# Posture Type One: Kyphosis and/or Lordosis

This posture type is very common. What has happened? Notice where the plumb line falls now:

- The head is thrust forward.

- The upper back, or thoracic spine, is overly rounded. A kyphosis just means a curvature, but in this case it would be more appropriate to talk about there being too much of a kyphosis.

- The shoulder blades are most probably abducted, that is, they have moved outward away from the ribcage.

- The pelvis is tilted forward, anteriorly rotated. Any change in the position of the pelvis will have an effect on the spine and the hips. In this case the spine has too much of a curve, it is overly hollowed, hyperextended.

- The hip joint is held in flexion.

- The knees are slightly hyperextended (locked back).

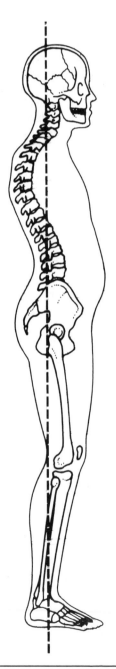

---

# Posture Type Two: The Swayback

This posture is often seen combined with the previous type, and is particularly popular among teenagers who have mastered the art of slouching.

- The head is forward of the plumb line.

- Shortened neck extensors.

- The deep neck flexors are lengthened.

- The thoracic spine has swayed noticeably backward.

- Thoracic back extensors are lengthened.

- Upper abdominals are shortened.

- The curvature of the lumbar spine is reduced, flattened.

- The pelvis is tilted backward, but moved slightly forward of the plumb line, meaning that the pelvis sways forward in relation to the feet.

- The hip joints are in extension.

- Hip flexors are lengthened.

- Gluteals are weak.

- Hamstrings are tight and short.

- Tensor fasciae latae are short.

- The knees are hyperextended (locked back).

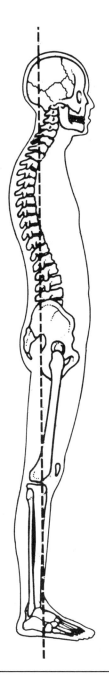

# Posture Type Three: The Flatback

This is relatively easy to spot since the back is flat.

- The head is again forward of the plumb line.

- Neck extensors are shortened.

- Deep neck flexors are lengthened.

- The thoracic area is interesting – the upper section can be rounded while the lower part is quite straight.

- Upper abdominals are short.

- There is a loss of the lumbar curve.

- Lower abdominals are weak.

- The pelvis is obviously tilted backward.

- Gluteus maximus and medius are weak.

- Hip flexors are lengthened.

- Hamstrings are short.

- Usually the knee joints are hyper-extended (locked back) but occasionally they can be held flexed.

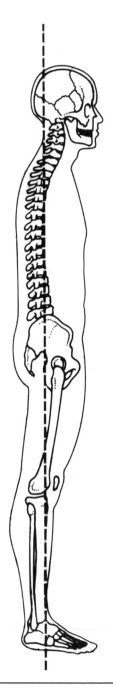

# Muscle Length Testing  Hamstring Test

Identifying your postural type is not always easy. Sometimes you are a combination of those shown. The best way to make sure which one you are is to stand in your underwear, your profile to a mirror, and get someone to hold a plumb line (a piece of string with a weight attached) and then compare this to the diagrams, noticing where the plumb line falls in relation to each postural type. But if you are in any doubt, consult your Pilates teacher or your medical practitioner for advice.

The other way to find out is to try testing the length of certain muscles such as the hamstrings or hip flexors, although we do not recommend this if you are in acute pain.

You will need to familiarize yourself with neutral alignment (page 62) before you attempt these tests. Later in the book we use very similar techniques to stretch these muscles if they do prove to be tight!

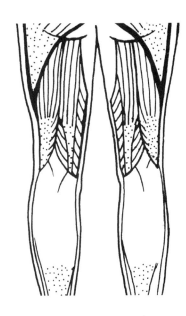

the hamstrings run along
the backs of both thighs

# Hamstring Test cont.

The hamstrings are, in fact, a group of three muscles, so called because in past times farmers would sever the hamstrings of pigs to prevent them from wandering away. The hamstrings flex and bend the knee. We spend far too much time sitting and, as a result, the hamstrings do not get the natural stretching they need. They can also become tight when they substitute for weak gluteal muscles.

If your hamstrings are too short, they will greatly restrict your flexibility and increase the risk of damage to the lumbar spine in everyday forward bending or sport. The length of the hamstring is determined by the straight-leg-raise test. Ideally you should find someone to help you to do this, but it is vital that the person who helps you does not pull hard on the leg or they will cause damage!

### Equipment
A scarf or stretch band, or a good friend.
A firm flat cushion (optional).

### Starting Position
- Lie on your back with your knees bent, hip-width apart and parallel. You may need a firm flat cushion under your head.
- If you are using the scarf, place it over the sole of one foot. If you have a friend helping, they can hold one leg (see photo) stretched out straight.

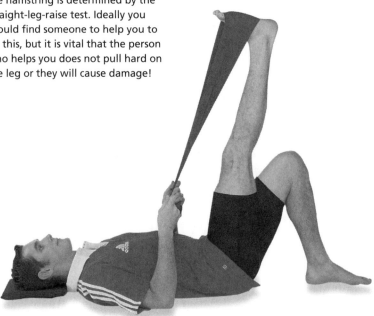

## Action

1 For the neutral position see the Compass on page 62.

2 Maintaining neutral "north to south" positioning, slowly straighten the leg into the air either with the help of the scarf or the friend.

3 Your tailbone stays down on the floor, you must keep neutral.

4 Notice how far you can straighten the leg before you lose the neutral pelvic position, that is, before your tailbone lifts and you lose the curve in your back (see below).

5 Relax the leg by gently bending it again.

6 Repeat on the other side.

By studying the chart below, you should be able to tell if your hamstrings are short. Please note that the opposite leg is stretched along the floor rather than bent at the knee (recommended in this test for beginners).

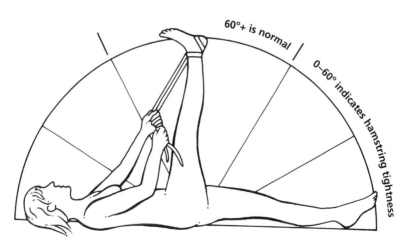

60°+ is normal

0–60° indicates hamstring tightness

# Hip Flexor Test (includes an iliotibial-band test)

## Equipment
A very sturdy table.
A firm flat cushion (optional).

## Starting Position
- Lie on your back at the edge of a sturdy table.
- Put a firm flat cushion under your head if you wish. Rest both feet on the edge of the table.

## Action
1 Take hold of your leg just above the knee and bend it, maintaining the spine and pelvis in neutral on the table (see the Compass page 62). Keep hold of the leg and keep it central.
2 Now, allow the other leg to slide gently off the table and hang down over the edge.
3 Make sure that your low back does not arch at all. It must remain flat/neutral.
4 Keep the lowered leg central, do not allow it to fall away to the side.
5 Check your alignment too – make sure that your pelvis is symmetrical and not twisted to one side.

**Good hip flexor length (normal)**

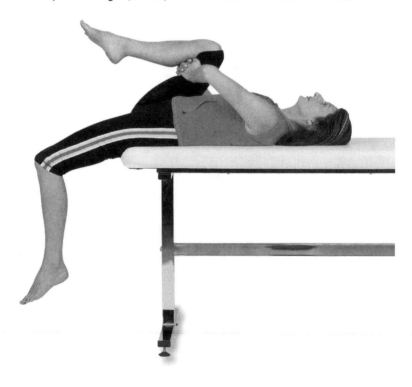

The length of the hip flexor is determined by the position of the leg over the edge of the table. It is considered tight if the knee is above hip-level to the horizontal plane. You can also see if the iliotibial band, which runs along the edge of your thighs, is tight. If it is, the leg will rest slightly out to the side, the kneecap facing outward. Repeat on the other side.

**Poor hip flexor length
(indicating hip flexors are shortened)**

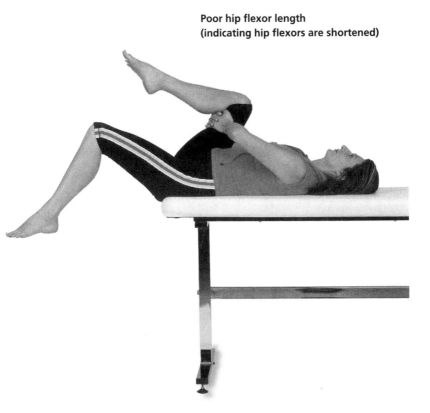

# How Do We Feel Pain?

This book has been written as a self-help manual for back-pain sufferers and for people who are interested in preventing back problems. What we obviously cannot do in a book of this nature is diagnose exactly what is wrong with you. For this, you need to see a medical practitioner who can properly examine and assess what is happening. At the end of this chapter, we will give you guidelines as to when it is advisable to seek help.

In the meantime, it is useful to look at different types of pain, how people describe their pain and how they actually feel pain. By doing this, you can better understand the nature of the problem and find a solution.

# Pain as a Sensation

All pain is unpleasant, but it is necessary for our survival because it is our warning signal that something is wrong. So, how do we feel it?

Pain is generated in the brain as a response to the pain receptors sending a signal to alert the brain that there is the threat of physical danger or disease. These signals are transmitted via the nerves. Remember that nerves are rather like electrical cables, they transmit impulses along nerve fibers. These sensory fibers transmit messages for the receptors in our skin, internal organs, muscles, ligaments and tendons. There are very few parts of the body that do not send pain signals.

**The control system: brain, spinal cord, spinal and peripheral nerves**

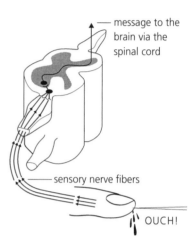

message to the brain via the spinal cord

sensory nerve fibers

OUCH!

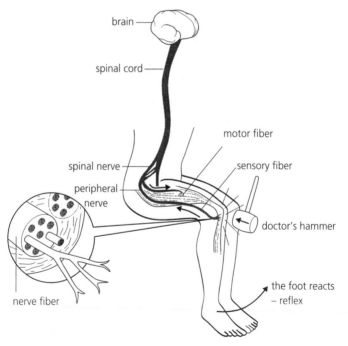

brain

spinal cord

motor fiber

spinal nerve

sensory fiber

peripheral nerve

doctor's hammer

the foot reacts – reflex

nerve fiber

# What Type of Pain Is It, and When Does It Occur?

This data, reproduced by kind permission of Peter O'Sullivan, shows the results of medical research he carried out in Australia in 1997 on how people described their pain:

Recurrent 70%
Constant 55%
Catching 45%
Locking 20%
Giving way 20%
Feeling of instability 35%

It appears then that most people describe back pain as being recurrent, that is, it keeps coming back. The next most common complaint is that the pain is constant, twenty-four hours a day, seven days a week without respite.

Other descriptions of back pain are:

- That it is "catching," implying that a particular movement causes the pain but that it switches off afterward.

- That it is "locking," suggesting that while undertaking a certain movement or activity the back gets stuck and refuses to move beyond that position.

- That they feel as though they are "giving way," in other words, there is the sensation that they have lost control of the movement.

- That there is a sense that sometimes the back is not stable, that it will not support them when they need it to.

In addition to noticing whether pain is constant, recurring and so on, you also need to decide if the pain is sharp or burning or a dull ache, or whether you may be feeling a tingling in your legs or have pins and needles. It is very helpful to your medical practitioner if you can decide which of these descriptions best explains your pain because it will help him or her in the assessment of your problem.

# How Bad Is the Pain?

Pain tends to be classified as either acute or chronic. Acute pain is a sudden, sharp sensation that warns us of immediate danger or threat to the body. Injuries like a burn or a cut are initially acute. Chronic pain is of a different nature. It is a dull pain, warning us of disease or the bad functioning of a part of the body rather than an immediate threat to the body's well-being.

Pain receptors send messages to the brain if stimulated to a certain degree. Furthermore, any state or event that causes the production of certain chemicals which change and sensitize the sensory organs will result in pain – for example, bruising, poor circulation or inflammation. When this happens, normal pain-free actions can become very painful because we are stretching or pressurizing sensitive nerves. This is important to remember when exercising, especially when stretching.

Pain intensifies not because the pain signal becomes stronger but because the frequency or number of pain messages increases. Usually acute pain blocks out chronic pain since the brain cannot receive both messages at once. The spinal cord will give priority to acute pain, the chronic pain only returning when the emergency is over. For example, that headache you have had all morning pales into the background when you stub your toe. Mother knew what she was doing when she "rubbed it better" because the sensation of rubbing the skin hard and fast "overrides" the pain underneath!

# Where Is the Pain Felt?

A back problem does not necessarily mean that you will feel pain in your back. The pain may be "referred." Referred pain can be described as occurring when you feel pain in one part of your body but the problem lies somewhere else. Common sites for pain caused by a back problem are:

- groin
- buttock
- abdomen
- leg
- foot
- pelvic floor

The first attack of mechanical back pain is usually felt in the center of the back or just to one side. Subsequent attacks may result in pain in the butt, the outside of the thigh as far down as the knee, or even below the knee to the ankle or foot. Referred pain from the back is less frequently felt in the front of the thigh. Some people may only feel pain in the legs and may never feel pain in the back at all.

**Common sites of back pain**

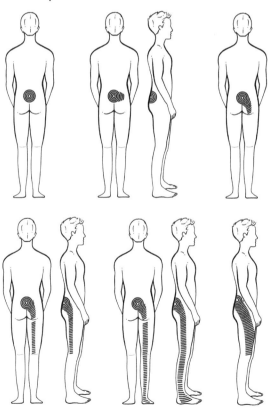

# When Should You Seek Emergency Medical Help?

**If your back pain is severe and linked with one of the following conditions or circumstances**, you should immediately ask someone to call a doctor or, in extreme cases, summon an ambulance. Try not to move.

- Call a doctor if you have been involved in a serious accident or had a bad fall. You might have seriously damaged your back and any movement might damage it further.
- You experience sudden numbness in one or both of your legs.
- You have pain in your chest or left arm.
- Your pain is growing worse and changing position does not help.
- Your pain is unbearable and there all the time.

- You have lost control over your bladder or bowels. This can be caused by a trapped nerve. Seeking medical advice as soon as possible will help to avoid permanent nerve damage.
- The pain awakens you at night. First you should look at how you are sleeping. See page 216 for advice on position. Should this not change your situation, seek medical advice to rule out infection.
- You experience weakness in your leg or you notice that the arch of a foot has dropped. This can be caused by a trapped nerve or a disc bulging, and needs prompt medical assessment.

You may find the following positions helpful in alleviating back pain that was not caused by an accident or a fall.

1 Lie on your side on a firm surface with your knees bent, keeping your spine and pelvis in neutral.
2 Try the Relaxation Position on page 61.
3 Try resting your feet on a chair as shown.

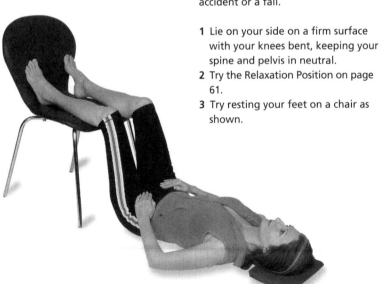

# How Body Control Pilates Can Help Back Problems

## Pain, Movement and Exercise

If you have suffered chronic pain for a long time you may be afraid to move, but movement is one way to help your problem. Welcome to the vicious circle!

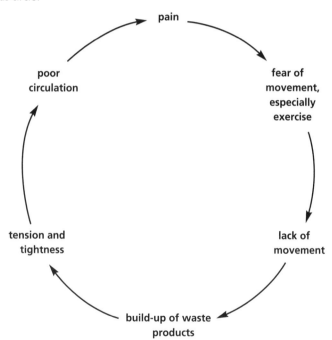

pain

fear of movement, especially exercise

lack of movement

build-up of waste products

tension and tightness

poor circulation

Perhaps you have suffered an injury or are experiencing pain and, as a result, you are afraid to move. The affected area may become inflamed. Perhaps you have muscle spasms, which make you even more tense and even more afraid to move.

The problem is that it is this very lack of movement that results in decreased local circulation, allowing waste products such as carbon dioxide and lactic acid to build up, thereby adding to the pain and so on.

One of the wonderful advantages of an exercise program such as Pilates is that the exercises are done slowly and with control. Your body will usually give you a warning signal if something is wrong so you can stop immediately, although this is not always the case because sometimes you may not feel pain after an inappropriate movement until some forty-eight hours later. However, we have designed the training program so that you add new movements one at a time and progressively. You may be advised to wait a couple of days after adding a new exercise just to be sure that it is appropriate.

As Pilates teachers, we have found that many of our clients have been in chronic pain for so long that they are afraid of movement. The sensory process (feedback from the receptors and the relevant response) may be altered. The gentle normal flowing movements involved in a Pilates session are a perfect way to reassure your body that it is okay to move again.

Before we move on to the main training program, let's take a closer method.

# The Eight Principles of Body Control Pilates

Body Control Pilates is more than just a set of exercises – it is a whole approach to movement. We have looked at all the reasons why most of us have lost the ability to move well. The aim of every Body Control Pilates exercise is to teach you how to move well again.

Eight Principles underlie all the exercises:

- Relaxation
- Concentration
- Alignment
- Breathing
- Centering
- Coordination
- Flowing Movements
- Stamina

# Relaxation

This is the starting point for everyone when they begin to learn Pilates. It may seem a strange way to begin an exercise routine to those of you more accustomed to jogging on the spot or stretching. Our first priority, however, is to ensure that you bring none of the stress of the day into your session. We have already seen how tense muscles are a major problem for people who suffer from back pain. Learning how to recognize and release areas of unwanted tension is a must before you work out, otherwise the wrong muscles will be firing up again and again and you'll never break the cycle of bad body use.

So where do most of us hold tension? The most common areas that tighten up are around the back of the neck and upper shoulders, places that you always want massaged. But if you sit a lot, you may also find the muscles around the front of the hips can get very tight. These hip flexor muscles can also shorten when there are faulty recruitment patterns. You may also feel tight in your lower back, especially if you have poor posture, and experience a lot of compression in the lumbar spine.

Our first goal in Pilates is, therefore, to teach you to be aware of tension and how to release it. The Relaxation Position on page 61 is a good way to start your session, allowing the stress of the day to melt away into the floor. You will also notice that we use this as the starting position for many of the exercises. Even when you advance in Pilates, however, you should be able to use this simple basic exercise to the same effect.

**The Relaxation Position**

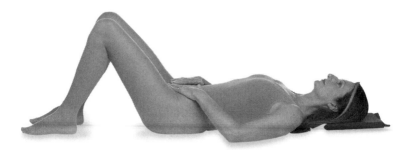

# Concentration

Remember: "It is the mind itself that builds the body."

Hopefully, you are now relaxed yet ready to begin to exercise. Another benefit that comes with relaxation is that it helps you to focus. Pilates is a mental and physical conditioning program, it aims to train both the mind and the body. You have already seen how movement takes place and noted the importance of constant input and output through neurological pathways to and from the brain: the two-way communication channel like a telephone connection. Just like a telephone, however, if there is no activity on the line for a long period, the chances are you'll get cut off! Pilates requires you to be constantly aware of how you are moving, and it requires you to focus your mind on each and every movement that you make. It develops your body's sensory feedback or proprioception, so that you know where you are in space and what you are doing with every part of your body. Although the movements themselves may become automatic with time, you still have to concentrate because there is always a further level of awareness to reach, layer adding on layer.

# Alignment

So now you are relaxed and focused. The next step is to bring the body into good postural alignment. By constantly reminding the body of how it should be standing, sitting or lying and by moving correctly you can gradually start to bring it back into proper alignment. This, as you have seen, is essential if you are going to restore the muscle balance in the body. If you exercise without due attention to the correct position of the joints, you risk stressing them and building imbalance into the surrounding muscles.

Good alignment of each and every part of the body while exercising is crucial to safety and to correcting muscle imbalances. You must have your bones in the right place to get the right muscles working. In that way, you build up the muscles so that they will support the joint, not stress it.

The Compass on page 62 is designed to help you find the correct neutral position of the pelvis and the spine. Once you are familiar with this in the Relaxation Position, you should practice finding neutral when standing, sitting and side-lying so that it becomes your normal position. Please note, though, that occasionally if the muscles around the pelvis are very out of balance, you may find neutral very difficult to maintain. When this is the case, we usually recommend that you consult your medical practitioner because it is often necessary to work in what is the best neutral you can achieve. Usually, after a few months, as the muscles begin to rebalance, true neutral becomes more comfortable. Nearly all our exercises should be performed in this neutral position unless you are told otherwise. You would not start your car if the gears were not in neutral, so please do not start an exercise unless you are in neutral!

**Neutral**

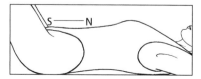

# Breathing

Hopefully, you are now relaxed, focused and aligned, so we need to concentrate next on improving the efficiency of your breathing. Stand in front of a mirror and watch the way you breathe. Take a deep breath. Notice what happens to your shoulders – do they rise up to your ears, accompanied by your heaving bosom (ladies only, of course)? Or perhaps your lower stomach expands when you breathe in? Both of these are inefficient ways of taking a breath.

So how do we want you to breathe? Wide and full into your back and sides. The ribcage should expand noticeably when you breathe in but most of us use just a fraction of this potential. By expanding the ribcage, the volume of the cavity is increased and the capacity for oxygen intake is therefore increased as well. It also encourages you to make maximum use of the lower part of your lungs. This type of breathing also works the muscles between the ribs, facilitating their expansion and making the upper body more fluid and mobile. We call it thoracic or lateral breathing. Your lungs become like bellows, the lower ribcage expanding wide as you breathe in and closing down as you breathe out. You do not want to block the descent of the diaphragm but, rather, encourage the movement to the sides and into the back.

The Lateral Breathing exercise on page 67 will help you to breathe laterally.

How you breathe is important to the Pilates method of exercising, as is the timing of the breath. You can help or hinder a movement by breathing in or out at the proper time. All Pilates exercises are carefully designed to reinforce and encourage the right muscle recruitment by using the breath correctly.

Most people find this timing difficult at first, especially if they are used to other fitness regimes, but once they have mastered this, it makes sense. As a general rule we:

- Breathe in to prepare for a movement and lengthen up through the spine.
- Breathe out, zip up from the pelvic floor and pull the lower abdominals toward the spine (see page 68), and move.
- Breathe in to recover, staying zipped up.

Moving on the exhalation will enable you to relax into the movement and prevent you from tensing. It also gives you greater core stability at the hardest part of the exercise and safeguards against you holding your breath, which can unduly stress the heart and lead to serious complications.

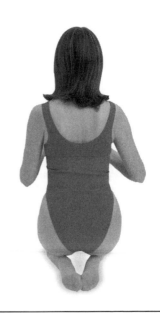

# Centering: Creating a "Girdle of Strength"

It is fascinating to think that, some ninety years ago, Joseph Pilates discovered that if he pulled his navel back toward his spine, his low back felt protected. He did not know this action gives you what physiotherapists call "core stability"; he simply had superb body awareness and thus introduced the direction "navel to spine" into all Pilates exercises.

We have already discussed, in the section on how the back works, the importance of the deep stabilizing muscles, especially transversus abdominis and multifidus. Just to give you an idea of how effective this natural corset of deep postural muscles can be, take a large towel and wind it tight around your middle. The support the towel gives you is a wonderful feeling, especially if you have back problems, and has the same effect as the deep stabilizing muscles.

We have had to adapt Joseph Pilates' original directions to incorporate the latest medical research, which indicates that the best

stability is to be achieved if the action begins with the pelvic floor and then the lower abdominals are engaged. This is why we now use the direction "zip up and hollow." As you breathe out, draw up the muscles of the pelvic floor and hollow the lower abdominals back to the spine as if you are zipping up this internal zipper. You will notice that we have chosen to use the word "hollow" to describe the action. It is very important that you do not grip your abdominals tightly because this will only create unnecessary tension and you will probably engage the wrong muscles to boot. Remember, stabilizing muscles need to be worked at less 30 percent of their full effort (MVC).

Once you have learned to create a strong center, you can then add movements such as rotation, extension and flexion. The exercises given on page 73 will take you through this step by step.

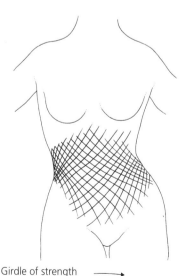

Girdle of strength

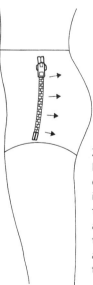

Zip up and hollow by drawing up and in the muscles of the pelvic floor and hollowing the lower abdomen back toward the spine

## Coordination

You have mastered lateral breathing, correct alignment and the creation of a strong center. You now need to learn how to add movement to the equation while maintaining this strong center. This is moving on to Stages 2 and 3 of the program. It is not easy to begin with but, like learning to drive a car, it soon becomes an automatic ("grooved") movement – a muscle memory. Meanwhile, the actual process of learning this coordination is excellent mental and physical training, stimulating that two-way communication channel. Remember that the brain remembers sequences of movements so you need to feed it good movement input, sound recruitment patterns.

We usually start with small movements and then build up to more complicated combinations. The idea is to challenge you constantly, to keep moving the goal posts. We may add resistance and load. Whatever exercise you are performing, however, the movements must be correctly executed with the right muscles doing the work, the right alignment, the right breathing. By repeating these sound movement patterns, we *can* start to change the way you move!

## Flowing Movements

Pilates is all about natural movements performed correctly, gracefully and with control. You will not be required to twist into any awkward positions or to strain. Movements are generally slow, lengthening away from the strong center. This gives you the opportunity to check your alignment and to focus on using the right muscles to do the job. You can also stop if you feel any discomfort, making Pilates one of the safest forms of exercise. Slow doesn't mean easy, though – in fact it is harder to do an exercise slowly than quickly, and it is also less easy to cheat!

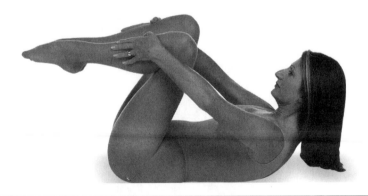

# Stamina

Slowly and gradually the Body Control Pilates program will start to build endurance into your muscles, especially the deep postural muscles. As you learn to move more efficiently and become more proficient at the exercises and your muscles begin to work the way nature intended, you will discover that your overall stamina improves dramatically. You will no longer be wasting energy holding on to unnecessary tension or moving inefficiently. Many people complain of tiredness after a day on their feet simply because standing badly is tiring: the ribcage is compressed and, as a consequence, the lungs are constricted. As you learn to open and lengthen the body, breathing becomes more efficient. All Pilates exercises are designed to encourage the respiratory, lymphatic and circulatory systems to function more effectively. Think of a well-serviced car in which the engine is tuned and the wheels aligned. It runs more efficiently, as will your body.

The only thing that Pilates doesn't offer is cardiovascular work. The importance of including some aerobic activity in your fitness program is now well known and you should aim to do three twenty-minute sessions a week to raise your heart rate.

Choosing a safe aerobic activity if you have a back problem is tricky because you must pick something that will not aggravate your back. You can consider brisk walking (but not power walking) or swimming – backstroke is especially suitable. Whichever activity; you choose, please bear in mind that you must use your body well while doing it or you will undo all the good you have done in your Pilates session.

Pilates is a great way of getting you fit for your chosen sport or activity, it ensures that you use your body correctly with sound movement patterns while you walk, run, play tennis or swim. It will help to prepare the body before your activity and rebalance it afterward.

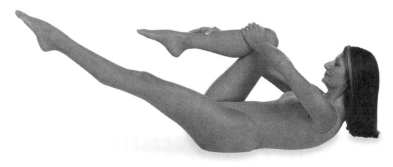

---

# The Body Control Pilates Back-Training Program

## *How to Use the Program*

Whether you are aiming to ease any discomfort you are experiencing in your back or you want to prevent the onset of back pain, you will need to follow gradual, progressive stages of training. The body needs time to change, strengthen and stretch. You are aiming to strengthen the muscles that support the spine and then ensure that they continue to work efficiently in order to prevent your back problem from returning.

The key message is to build up your training program gradually. Be careful not to add too many new movements in one session. It is advisable to wait a few days after adding a new exercise to see if it is suitable for you. If you experience any discomfort, leave that movement out because you may not be ready for it. Remember, there are no quick fixes! It is going to take time and a level of commitment to achieve success.

On pages 187–210 we have given you lots of different workouts of different lengths and levels to try. Anyone with a back problem should aim to do at least fifteen minutes of Pilates per day without fail. Then, on days when you have more time, you can add extra exercises.

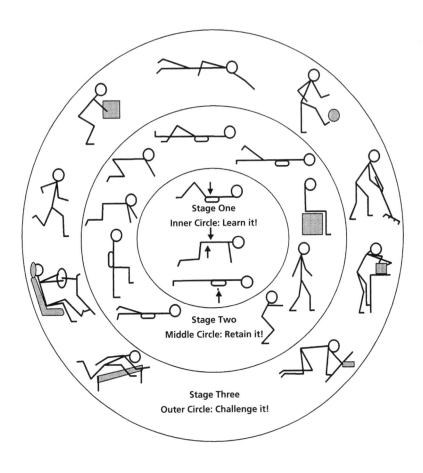

Stage One
Inner Circle: Learn it!

Stage Two
Middle Circle: Retain it!

Stage Three
Outer Circle: Challenge it!

The Body Control Pilates back-training program
consists of a circle of three concentric rings

# Stage One Inner Circle: Learn It!

You will start your exercise program with the exercises in the inner ring. This is Stage One – the learning stage that incorporates the initial principles of Relaxation, Concentration, Alignment, Breathing and Centering. The exercises here are designed to work on your body awareness, which will help you to learn good body alignment, in particular the neutral position of the pelvis and spine. You will learn how to locate, activate and strengthen the deep stabilizing muscles (transversus abdominis, pelvic floor, multifidus). Finally, you will learn how to breathe laterally and efficiently. With your improved body awareness, you will be able to move with good muscle recruitment and without the substitution of the superficial mobilizing muscles.

All the exercises in this section have this symbol 🐾 that indicates this level.

The Relaxation Position
The Compass
The Compass against the Wall
Alignment in Standing
Lateral Breathing
The Pelvic Elevator
Stabilizing on All Fours
Stabilizing in Prone-lying
Stabilizing in the Relaxation Position
Pelvic Stability Exercises: Leg Slides, Knee Drops, Knee Folds and Turning out the Leg
The Dart: Stage One
Floating Arms
Scapular Awareness Exercise against the Wall
The Starfish
Neck Rolls and Chin Tucks
Shoulder Drops

# Stage Two  Middle Circle: Retain It!

Once you have mastered Stage One, you may progress to Stage Two, which involves practicing the skills you have learned again and again, until the pattern of movement is locked or grooved into your memory banks. You are now moving on to the principles of Coordination, Flowing Movements and Stamina, while still incorporating the basic principles of Relaxation, Concentration, Alignment, Breathing and Centering. The beauty of the Body Control Pilates method is that it will not feel as if you are doing hundreds of repetitions because the exercises are designed to complement each other. You will learn now to refine these newly learned skills, maintaining the stabilizers, keeping correct alignment and control. At this stage you add segmental control, which is moving the spine vertebra by vertebra like a wheel, and also rotation.

All the exercises in this section have this symbol 🖐 that indicates this level.

Spine Curls
Hip Flexor Stretch
Side Rolls
Knee Circles with Breath
Windmill Arms
Walking on the Spot plus Calf Stretch
Arm Circles against the Wall
Arm Circles: Free Standing
Side Reach against the Wall
Dumb Waiter on the Wall
Knee Swings
The Oyster
The Big Squeeze
The Star
The Rest Position: Two Versions
Curl Ups
Oblique Curl Ups
Hamstring Stretch
Adductor Openings
Wide Leg Stretch against the Wall
Chicken Wings on the Wall
Floating Arms against the Wall
Sitting Waist Twists
Standing Waist Twists
Standing on One Leg
Table Top: Stages One and Two
The Diamond Press
The Dart: Stage Two
Ankle Circles
Foot Exercises
Deep Gluteal Stretch against the Wall
The Monkey
The Cat
Side-lying Quadriceps and Hip Flexor Stretch
Arm Openings
The Cushion Squeeze

# Stage Three  Outer Circle: Challenge It!

Now you're cooking! This section includes many classic Pilates exercises, which are complex choreographed sequences. You can also add load or perhaps vary the starting position of an exercise to make it more challenging. You should still continue to include exercises from the first two stages.

All the exercises in this section have this symbol  that indicates this level.

The Pelvic Bridge
Roll Downs
Hip Rolls with Shoulder Blade Setting
Butt Scrunches
Full Table Top
The Torpedo
One-legged Calf Raises
Abductor Lifts
Adductor Lifts
Inner-thigh Toner
Backstroke Swimming
Single Leg Stretch
The Hundred (Stages One to Four)

# Before You Begin . . .

- Be sure that you have no pressing unfinished business.
- Take the telephone off the hook, or put the answering machine on.
- You may prefer silence, otherwise put on some unobtrusive classical or new-age music.
- All exercises should be done on a padded mat.
- Wear something warm and comfortable that allows free movement.
- Barefoot is best, socks otherwise.
- The best time to exercise is in the late afternoon or evening when your muscles are already warmed up as a result of the day's activity. Exercising in the morning is fine, but you will need to take longer to warm up thoroughly.
- You will need space to work in – you cannot keep stopping to move furniture. Some clear wall space will be needed if you are going to do wall exercises.
- Items you may need include: a chair; a small flat but firm cushion for behind your head or perhaps a folded towel; a larger cushion; a long scarf and a tennis ball.

Please do not exercise if:

- You are feeling unwell.
- You have just eaten a heavy meal.
- You have been drinking alcohol.
- You are in pain from an injury – always consult your medical practitioner first because rest may be needed before you exercise.
- You have taken pain killers – they will mask any warning pains.
- You are undergoing medical treatment, or are taking drugs – again, you will need to consult your medical practitioner first.

And please remember that:

- Not all the exercises are suitable if you are pregnant.
- It is always wise to consult your doctor before taking up a new exercise regime.
- If you have a back problem you will need to consult your medical practitioner before starting this program. Many of the exercises are wonderful for back-related problems, but you should always seek expert guidance.

# Stage One

# Inner Circle: Learn it!

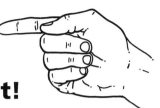

# The Relaxation Position

## Aim

To prepare the mind and body for exercise. To be used as a starting and finishing position for exercises and at the end of a session to unwind. To release unwanted tension from the body, allowing the torso to widen and the spine to lengthen.

## Equipment

A small flat firm cushion (optional).

## Starting Position

• Lie on your back on a mat. You may need a small firm flat cushion under your head to allow your neck to maintain its natural curve and stay lengthened and released. You should feel very comfortable.

• Bend your knees and place your feet flat on the floor in line with your hips. Some people are more comfortable with them placed a little wider, in line with the shoulders. This is fine.

• Keep your feet parallel to each other.

• Think of three points – the base of the big toe, the base of the small toe and the center of the heel. Keep your weight evenly balanced on these three points.

• Place your hands on your lower abdomen.

## Action

1 Allow your whole body to widen and lengthen.
2 Notice any areas of tension and allow them to melt gently into the floor.
3 Imagine you have dry sand in your back pockets. Allow it to trickle slowly out of your pockets on to the floor.
4 Release your thighs and soften the area around your hips.
5 Release your neck.

### Variations

You could also try this exercise with your feet up on a chair, which will help your low back muscles to release.

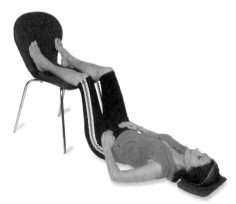

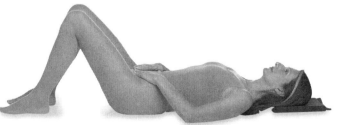

# The Compass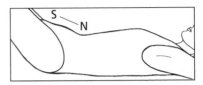

## Aim
To find the neutral position of the pelvis and spine.

## Equipment
A small flat firm cushion (optional).

## Starting Position
- Lie on your back in the Relaxation Position, with your head on the cushion if it makes you more comfortable. Imagine that you have a compass on your lower abdomen: the navel is north, the pubic bone south, with west and east on either side.

**Tilted to north**

## Action
1 First you will try two incorrect positions in order to find the correct one. Tilt your pelvis up toward north – while doing so, the pelvis will "tuck under." Notice what has happened to your waist, your hips and your tailbone. The waist is flattened – you've pushed it into the floor – and the curve in the back is lost. You have gripped the muscles around your hips and your tailbone has lifted off the floor.

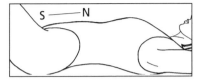

**Tilted to south**

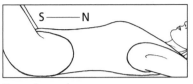

**Neutral**

**2** Now, carefully and gently (avoid this part if you have a back injury) position the pelvis so that it is tilting down toward south. Notice again what has happened. The low back is arched and feels vulnerable, your ribs have flared, you probably have two chins and your stomach is sticking out.

**3** Come back to the Starting Position.

**4** You are aiming for a neutral position between these two extremes, neither too north nor south, neither tucked nor arched. Back to the image of the compass: the pointer is level like a spirit level. The tailbone remains down on the floor and lengthens away. The pelvis keeps its length and is not "scrunched up" at all. There remains a small natural arch in your back. This is neutral, and all the exercises should be performed in this neutral position unless you are told other-wise. You should learn to recognize your natural neutral position in standing, lying, sitting, side-lying. As we like to remind you, you would not start your car if the gears were not in neutral, so please do not start an exercise unless you are in neutral!

**5** Be particularly vigilant when you are engaging the lower abdominals because there is then the temptation to tilt or tuck the pelvis. If you are lying down, you can always try placing your hand under your waist – you can feel if you are pushing the spine into the floor. You want to avoid this.

**NOTE** It is also worth pointing out that if you have a large butt, you will have more of a hollow in the lumbar region – this does not necessarily mean that you have arched your back. Learn to recognize your natural curve.

# The Compass against the Wall

You can also do the Compass lying down.

## Starting Position

- Stand with your feet about eight inches away from the wall and then lean back into it; your knees will be bent as if you are sitting on a high bar stool.
- Do not tip your head back to make it touch the wall, but lengthen up through the top of the head.
- Notice which parts of your back naturally touch the wall.

## Action

1 Gently tilt your pelvis to the north, so that your tailbone lifts away from the wall and the small of your back has flattened into it; the natural curve of your spine is lost.

2 Now gently and very slowly tilt your pelvis to the south (avoid this if you have a back injury). Feel the hollow of your back increase.

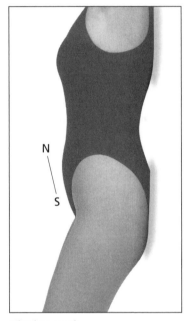

**Tilted to south**

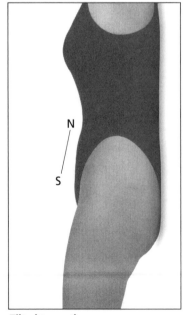

**Tilted to north**

**3** Try to find the mid-point between north and south so that the pubic bone and the prominent bones of your pelvis are level vertically. There should be a natural curve in your back and your tailbone should remain on the wall. Your ribs should not be flared. This is neutral.

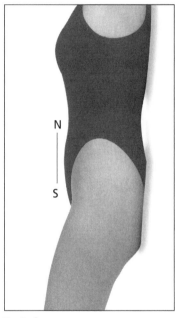

**Neutral**

Bear in mind that you also want the pelvis to be level "west to east." Many people suffer from a twisted pelvis; it can be rotated forward on one side as well as tilted. You need to be constantly aware that the pelvis must stay neutral, level and stable while you exercise if the right muscles are to work. Of course, once we add movements into the program the pelvis will sometimes move out of neutral, for example, in Roll Downs.

Please note that, occasionally, if the muscles around the pelvis are very out of balance, you may find neutral very difficult to maintain. When this is the case, we usually recommend that you consult your medical practitioner because it is often necessary to work in whatever is the best neutral you can achieve. Usually, after a few months, as the muscles begin to rebalance, neutral becomes more comfortable.

# Alignment in Standing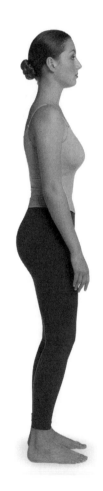

## Aim

To learn good alignment in standing.

In the last two exercises you had the floor and the wall to help you find your neutral pelvis and spinal positions. It is harder to find them without these aids to guide you, but the directions given below should help.

- Allow your head to go forward and up.

- Allow your neck to release.

- Keep your shoulder blades down your back.

- Keep your breastbone soft.

- Allow your elbows to open.

- Lengthen up through the spine.

- Check your pelvis – is it in neutral?

- Release your knees.

- What about your feet and legs? Usually, they should be hip-width apart and parallel.

- Keep the weight even on both feet – do not allow them to roll in or out.

  Think of three points on the soles of your feet – the base of your big toe, the base of your little toe and the center of your heel. These points form a triangle; keep the weight even on these three points.

# Lateral Breathing

## Aim

With thoracic or lateral breathing, your lungs become like bellows, the lower ribcage expanding wide as you breathe in and closing down as you breathe out. This type of breathing encourages correct movement patterns by enabling you to stay centered while you move. To practice try the following:

## Action

**1** Stand as per the directions in the last exercise. Wrap a scarf or towel around your ribs, crossing it over at the front.

**2** Holding the ends of the scarf or towel and gently tightening it, breathe in and allow your ribs to expand into it. As you breathe out, you can gently pull the ends of the scarf or towel together to help you fully empty your lungs. Relax the ribcage and allow the breastbone to soften. Watch that you do not lift the breastbone too high.

**3** Breathe easily and naturally. As you breathe in you might like to think of your ribs moving like an umbrella opening, as you breathe out the umbrella closes.

**4** Practice about ten breaths at a time and then take a break. Sometimes you can feel quite dizzy with this type of breathing simply from the extra intake of oxygen. Just stop for a while and start again when you feel better.

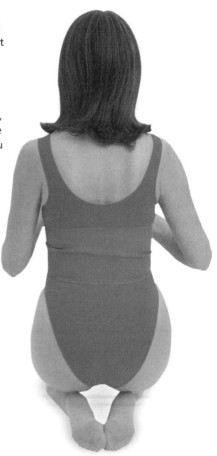

# The Pelvic Elevator

## Aim

To isolate and engage the deep stabilizing muscles of the pelvis and the spine: transversus abdominis, pelvic floor and multifidus.

In order to achieve the best possible stability, you need to be able to contract the pelvic floor at the same time as hollowing the lower abdominals to engage the transversus abdominis. It is not easy to isolate and engage the pelvic floor and it takes considerable concentration. We are talking about the urethra in men and women and the muscles of the vagina for women. At this stage, we do not want you to engage the muscles around the anus because it is too easy for the butt muscles to kick in and substitute. Think of a camera shutter closing and try to close it from side to side rather than front to back. It sounds weird, but one way to help locate the pelvic floor muscles is to suck your thumb as you draw them up inside. Crazy, but effective. Guys, you should think about lifting your "crown jewels."

Once you have found the pelvic floor muscles, it should be easier to isolate the transversus abdominis. To engage the transversus correctly (at no more than 25 percent MVC) think of:

- hollowing
- scooping
- drawing back the abdominals toward the spine
- sucking in

## Starting Position

- Sit on an upright chair.
- Make sure that you are sitting square with your weight even on both butt cheeks.
- Imagine that your pelvic floor is like the elevator in a building. This exercise requires you to take the "elevator" up to different floors.

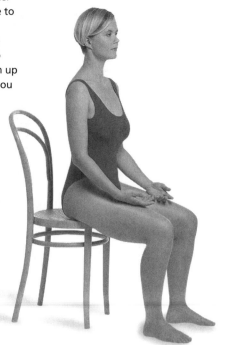

## Action

1 Breathe in, wide and full, into your back and sides and lengthen up through the spine.

2 As you breathe out, draw together the muscles of the pelvic floor, as if you are trying to prevent the flow of urine, and take the pelvic elevator up to the first floor of the building.

3 Breathe in and release the elevator back to the ground floor.

4 Breathe out and now take the elevator up to the second floor of the building.

5 Breathe in and release.

6 Breathe out and take the elevator up to the third floor, around about your navel.

7 Breathe in and relax.

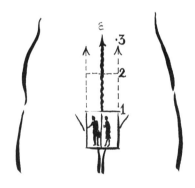

Try the same exercise, but this time place your hands on your lower abdomen. Notice at which point your lower abdominals hollow – most people feel some abdominal hollowing between the first and second floor. This is perfect recruitment as it keeps the action low and gentle. Think about what happened when you took the elevator to the top floor. When you do this your rectus abdominis muscle (the "six-pack" muscle) kicks in, dominating the action, so that the transversus does not engage – this is a wrong recruitment. By starting the action from underneath, you  the six-pack muscle to stay quiet.

**Remember, when engaging the stabilizing muscles, you want to start the action from the pelvic floor, draw the muscles together like sliding doors then take them just a little way up inside until you reach no higher than the second floor, just until you feel your lower abdominals hollow. From now on we will refer to this as "zipping up and hollowing."**

### Watchpoints

• Do not allow the butt muscles to join in.
• Keep your jaw relaxed.
• Don't take your shoulders up to the top floor too; keep them down and relaxed.
• Try not to grip around your hips.
• Keep the pelvis and spine quite still.

**Once you have found your pelvic floor muscles, you need to learn how to engage them in lots of different positions. You also need to learn how to keep them engaged for both the in and out breaths.**

# Stabilizing on All Fours

## Aim
To locate the deep stabilizing muscles.

## Starting Position
- Kneel on all fours, your hands beneath your shoulders, shoulder-width apart, fingers facing forward.
- Make sure you haven't locked your elbows, keep them soft. Your knees are beneath your hips.
- Have the top of your head lengthening away from your tailbone.
- Your pelvis is in its neutral position. It helps to think of a small pool of water sitting in the small of your back.
- Let your abdominals relax.

## Action
1 Breathe in, wide and full, to prepare.
2 Breathe out, and zip up and hollow the lower abdominals toward the spine. Your back should not move at all. Remember to keep the action low and gentle.
3 Breathe in and release.
4 Once you are happy that you can isolate the right muscles, try to hold the zip up and hollow while you breathe in and out. Breathe laterally – wide and full – so you are not tempted to use the wrong muscles. Work up to holding the zip up and hollow for ten seconds.
5 This may sound a little strange, but try this exercise in your underwear with a mirror placed on the mat below your stomach – pull the curtains first, though! Use the mirror to check that you keep the action low and gentle. You want to avoid the six-pack muscle kicking in.

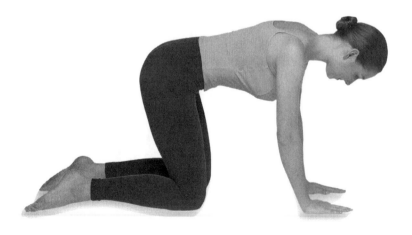

# Stabilizing in Prone-lying

## Equipment
A small flat firm cushion (optional).

## Starting Position
- Lie on your front. Rest your forehead on your folded hands, open the shoulders out and relax the upper back – you may need a small, flat cushion under your abdomen if your low back is uncomfortable.
- Your legs are shoulder-width apart and relaxed.

## Action
1 Breathe in, wide and full.
2 Breathe out, zip up from the pelvic floor and lift your lower abdominals off the floor. Imagine there is a precious egg under them that must not be crushed. Do not tighten the butt.
3 Breathe in and release.
4 There should be no movement in the pelvis or spine.
5 Once you are happy that you have found the right muscles, work up to holding the zip up and hollow for your in and out breath for ten seconds.
6 Repeat ten times.

# Stabilizing in the Relaxation Position

## Equipment
A small flat firm cushion (optional).

## Starting Position
- Lie on your back in the Relaxation Position, with your head on the cushion if it makes you more comfortable, and check that your pelvis is in neutral.
- Place your hands on your pelvis. Find your prominent pelvic bones (anterior superior iliac spines). Put your fingertips on these bones then move them about one inch inward and one inch downward. Very, very gently feel your deep abdominals in their relaxed state. Do not do this if you have abdominal problems or if it causes you discomfort.

## Action
1 Breathe in, wide and full, to prepare.
2 Breathe out and zip up and hollow.
3 You should feel the deep muscles under your fingers engage and become firm, rather as if an airplane seat belt was being wrapped around you. If the muscles are recruited correctly they will stay scooped and not bulge out at all.
4 Do not allow the pelvis to tuck under. Do not push into the spine.

Keep your tailbone on the floor and lengthening away.
5 Now, breathe laterally into your sides and back as you hold the zip up and hollow for up to a count of ten. Then relax.

## Watchpoints
- You must be careful not to tuck the pelvis under, that is, tilting it north. If you do, you will lose your neutral position and it means that other muscles – the rectus abdominis and hip flexors – are cheating and doing the work instead of the transversus abdominis and internal obliques.
- Once you have learned to create a strong center, you can then add movements such as rotation, flexion, extension. The exercises given on page 73 will take you through this step by step.

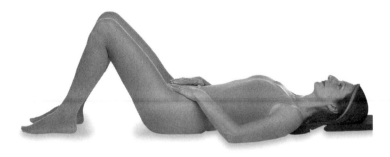

# Pelvic Stability Exercises: Leg Slides, Knee Drops, Knee Folds and Turning out the Leg

You are now going to try a variety of movements to check that the lumbar spine and pelvis can stay stable.

## Aim

To learn how to keep the pelvis and lumbar spine neutral and stable while the limbs are moved.

Now that you have mastered the breathing, the correct alignment of the pelvis and the spine and how to engage the deep stabilizing muscles, you need to learn how to add movement and to coordinate all this. It isn't easy to begin with but, as with learning to ride a bicycle, it soon becomes automatic. Meanwhile, the process of learning this coordination is fabulous mental and physical training since it stimulates that two-way communication between the brain and the muscles – real mind-body exercises.

We usually start with small, simple movements and then build up to more complicated combinations. Here, we have given you four exercises to practice, all of them requiring you to keep the pelvis and lumbar spine completely still. A useful image to keep in mind is of a set of car headlights sitting on your pelvis shining at the ceiling. The beam should be fixed and not mimicking searchlights. You can vary which exercises you practice at each session. The Starting Position is the same for all three.

## Equipment for All Pelvic Stability Exercises

A small flat firm cushion (optional).

## Starting Position for All Pelvic Stability Exercises

- Lie in the Relaxation Position with your head on the cushion.
- Check that your pelvis is in neutral, tailbone down and lengthening away.
- Place your hands on your pelvic bones to check for unwanted movement.

## Action for Leg Slides

1 Breathe in, wide and full, to prepare.

2 Breathe out, zip up and hollow and slide one leg away along the floor, keeping the lower abdominals engaged and the pelvis still, stable and in neutral.

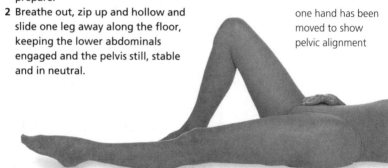

one hand has been moved to show pelvic alignment

3 Breathe into your lower ribcage while you return the leg to the bent position, at the same time trying to keep the stomach hollow. If you cannot yet breathe in and maintain a strong center, then take an extra breath and return the leg on the out breath.

4 Repeat five times with each leg.

## Action for Knee Drops

1 Breathe in, wide and full, to prepare.
2 Breathe out, zip up and hollow and allow one knee to open slowly to the side. Go only as far as the pelvis stays still.

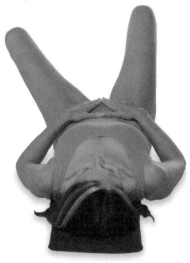

3 Breathe in, still zipped and hollowed, and return the knee to the center.
4 Repeat five times with each leg.

## Action for Knee Folds

With this movement it is particularly useful to feel that the abdominal muscles stay "scooped" and do not bulge while you fold the knee in, so you may like to find your pelvic bones again and move your fingers about one inch inward and two inches downward. Very gently feel the muscles engage as you zip up and hollow.

1 Breathe in, wide and full, to prepare.
2 Breathe out, zip up and hollow and fold the right knee up. Think of the thigh bone dropping down into the hip and anchoring there. Do not lose your neutral pelvis. The tailbone stays down. Do not rely on the other leg to stabilize you. Imagine that your foot is on a large chocolate eclair; you don't want to press down on it.

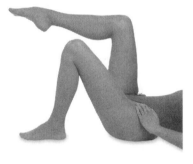

3 Feel with your fingers that your lower abdominals have stayed scooped and have not bulged out or thickened.
4 Breathe in and hold.
5 Breathe out and stay zipped and hollowed as you slowly return the foot to the floor.
6 Repeat five times with each leg.

If you find it difficult to lift the leg while keeping your lower abdominals hollow, imagine that you are slowly lifting the foot off a set of bathroom scales. You can then gradually build up to lifting the foot fully off the scales.

## Action for Turning out the Leg

This next action involves turning the leg out from the hip. As you do so, you are working your deep gluteal muscles, especially gluteus medius, which is one of the main stabilizing muscles of the pelvis.

**Please seek advice if you suffer from sciatica.**

1 Follow Steps 1 and 2 for Knee Folds.
2 Breathe out, zip up and hollow and turn the right leg out from the hip, bringing the foot up to touch the left knee if you can.
3 Do not allow the pelvis to tilt, twist or turn; keep it central and stable. Remember, headlights glued to the ceiling!
4 Breathe in and then out, and zip up and hollow as you reverse the movement to return the foot to the floor.
5 Repeat five times on each side.

## Watchpoints

• Remember that you are trying to avoid even the slightest movement of the pelvis.
• It helps to think of the waist being long and even on both sides as you make the movement.
• Try to keep your neck and jaw released throughout. If you feel tension creeping in, do a few Neck Rolls and Chin Tucks (page 84).

### Useful Tip

A useful way of checking that you are stabilizing correctly is to place your hands, palms down, under your waist. As you zip up and hollow you may feel your muscles engage but you should not be pushing into your hands. You can then feel if there is any unwanted change in pressure as you slide, drop or fold the leg.

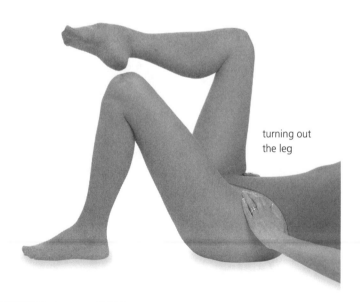

turning out
the leg

# The Dart: Stage One

The final part of the "girdle of strength" involves learning how to stabilize the shoulder blades. You have been concentrating on the lower half of the body but you also need to learn how to move the upper body correctly with good mechanics. For this, you need to find the muscles (lower trapezius and serratus anterior) that set the shoulder blades down into the back, holding them in just the right position to allow the arms to move freely and easily, with the shoulder joints correctly positioned.

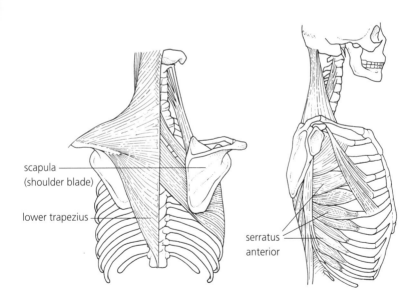

scapula (shoulder blade)

lower trapezius

serratus anterior

## Aim

To locate the muscles that stabilize the shoulder blades.

## Equipment

Two firm flat cushions (optional).

### Starting Position

- Lie on your front.
- You can place a cushion under your forehead to allow you to breathe more easily if you'd like.
- If it makes you more comfortable you can also put a cushion underneath your stomach.
- Have your arms down by your sides, your palms facing the ceiling.
- Your neck is long.
- Your legs are relaxed but parallel.

## Action

1 Breathe in, wide and full, to prepare and lengthen through the spine, tucking your chin in gently.
2 Breathe out, zip up and hollow – stay zipped and hollowed throughout the exercise – and pull your shoulder blades down into your back.
3 Turn your palms to face your body, and reach your fingers toward your feet. The top of your head stays lengthening away from you.
4 Keep looking straight down at the floor. Do not tip your head back.
5 Breathe in and feel the length of your body from the tips of your toes to the top of your head.
6 Breathe out and release.

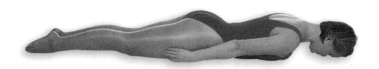

## Watchpoints

- Keep hollowing the lower abdominals.
- Do not strain the neck; it should feel released as your shoulders engage down into your back. Think of a swan's neck extending out from between its wings.
- Remember to keep your feet on the floor.
- Please stop if you feel at all uncomfortable in the low back.
- This exercise can also be done with the feet hip-width apart and the thigh and butt muscles relaxed.

# Floating Arms

The muscles that you felt pulling your shoulder blades down into your back in the Dart are the stabilizing muscles. Now that you have located them, try to feel them working in this next exercise.

**Aim**

To learn correct upper-body mechanics.

**Starting Position**

- Stand correctly as discussed in Alignment in Standing on page 66.
- Now, place your right hand on your left shoulder, on the muscle that tends to become tight when you are stressed. The idea is that your hand checks that this muscle, which is the upper part of your trapezius muscle, remains "quiet" for as long as possible. Very often this part will overwork, so think of it staying soft and released, while the lower trapezius below your shoulder blades works to set your shoulders down into your back.

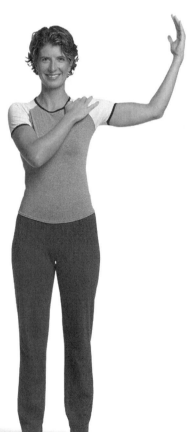

## Action

1 Breathe in to prepare and lengthen up through the spine, letting the neck be free.

2 Breathe out, zip up and hollow and slowly begin to raise your left arm, with your palm facing the floor, reaching wide out of the shoulder blade like a bird's wing. Think of the hand leading the arm and the arm following the hand as it floats upward.

## Watchpoints

• Keep a sense of openness in the upper body.
• Do not allow your upper body to shift to the side, keep centered.

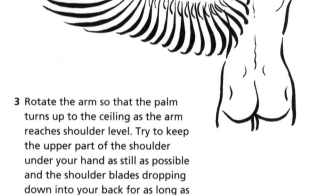

3 Rotate the arm so that the palm turns up to the ceiling as the arm reaches shoulder level. Try to keep the upper part of the shoulder under your hand as still as possible and the shoulder blades dropping down into your back for as long as possible.

4 Breathe in as you lower your arm to your side. Repeat three times with each arm.

# Scapular Awareness Exercise against the Wall

### Aim
To identify the lower trapezius muscles used to stabilize the shoulder blades.

Here is one final exercise to help you isolate these important muscles. Use what you have learned in the last two exercises.

### Starting Position
- Stand facing a wall with your toes several inches away from it, feet hip-width apart and parallel. Make sure that your knees are soft.
- Raise your arms above you wider than shoulder-width apart, palms facing each other, the edge of your hands against the wall. Your thumbs will therefore point away from the wall.

### Action
1 Breathe in, wide and full, and lengthen through the spine.
2 Breathe out, zip up and hollow – stay zipped and hollowed throughout the exercise – and draw your shoulder blades down toward the small of your back.
3 Breathe in and hold.
4 Breathe out and release.

### Watchpoints
- Keep your neck released.
- Keep your upper body open.
- Keep lengthening up through the top of your head. Do not be tempted to lean forward into the wall or back away from it.
- Stay centered.

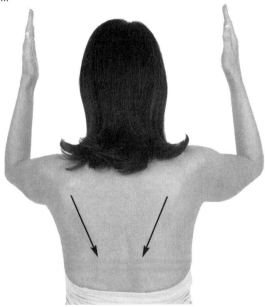

# The Starfish

## Stage One: The Upper Body

Now you can combine everything you have learned.

### Equipment
A flat firm cushion (optional).

### Starting Position
• Lie in the Relaxation Position, with your arms down by your sides, and your head on the cushion if it makes you more comfortable.

### Action
1 Breathe in wide into your lower ribcage to prepare.
2 Breathe out, zip up and hollow and start to take one arm back as if to touch the floor. If you cannot touch the floor easily, only take the arm as far back as is comfortable. On no account force it backward, keep it soft and open with the elbow bent. Your shoulder blade stays down into your back. Your ribs stay calm and do not flare up. Do not allow your back to arch at all.
3 Breathe in as you return the arm to your side. Repeat five times with each arm.
4 Not everyone can touch the floor in this position without arching the upper back. Do not strain. It is better to keep the back down than force the arm down.

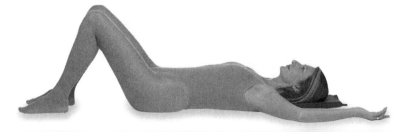

# Stage Two: The Full Starfish

Now you are going to coordinate the opposite arm and leg movement away from your strong center. Although this looks simple, it is a sophisticated movement pattern, using all the skills of good movement you have learned so far. It is the base on which you will build your whole fitness program.

### Equipment and Starting Position
Same as Stage One.

### Action
1 Breathe in, wide and full, to prepare.
2 Breathe out, zip up and hollow – stay zipped and hollowed throughout the exercise. Slide the right leg away along the floor, at the same time taking the left arm above you in a backstroke movement.
3 Keep the pelvis completely neutral, stable and still, and the stomach muscles engaged.
4 Keep a sense of width and openness in the upper body and shoulders, and try to keep the shoulder blades down into your back, the ribs calm.
5 Breathe in and return the limbs to the Starting Position.
6 Repeat five times, alternating arms and legs.

### Watchpoints
- Do not be tempted to overreach, the girdle of strength must stay in place.
- Slide the leg in a line with the hip.

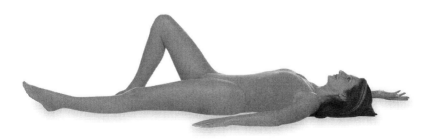

# Neck Rolls and Chin Tucks

### Aim

To become aware of, and learn to release, tension accumulated in the neck. To use the deep stabilizers in the neck and to stretch the neck extensors, which tilt the head back, gently.

The neck is an important part of the spine. It allows great mobility and has to support a relatively heavy head. Problems in the back will quite often cause pain and discomfort in the neck.

### Equipment

One or two firm flat cushions.

### Starting Position

- Lie in the Relaxation Position with the hands resting on the lower abdomen.
- Your head should rest on a firm flat cushion. Make sure the cushion is not under the neck.
- Sometimes more than one cushion is needed to fully relax the neck and chest.

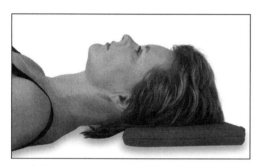

Good alignment

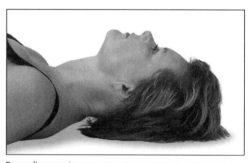

Poor alignment

## Action

1 Relax your neck and jaw. Allow your tongue to widen at its base. The back of your neck should stay long.

2 Release your breastbone and let the shoulder blades sink into the floor. The chest opens.

3 Let your head roll *slowly* to one side. It is important not to force this movement so you are still able to relax.

4 Bring the head back to the center and gently let it roll to the other side. Take your time.

5 Try to notice if there is a difference between the two sides.

6 After four repetitions bring your head to the center and gently tuck your chin in, keeping the head on the floor and lengthening out of the back of the neck. It is a subtle movement – imagine you have a ripe peach under your chin that you want to hold but not crush its delicate skin.

7 Return the head to the Starting Position.

8 Repeat the rolling to the side and chin tucks eight times.

## Watchpoints

• Keep the movement smooth and do not force the head.

• Try to roll the head directly to the side, rotating it around its central axis.

• When tucking the chin, the head remains on the floor.

• The jaw stays released throughout.

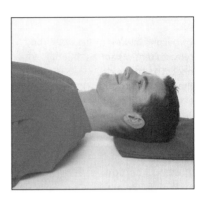

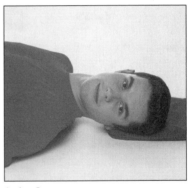

Action 3

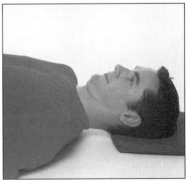

Action 6

# Shoulder Drops

## Aim
To release tension in the upper body.

A wonderful exercise that allows you to let go of any tension in the shoulders and neck. Great to do at the end of a stress-filled day.

## Equipment
A firm flat cushion (optional).

## Starting Position
• Lie in the Relaxation Position, with your head on the cushion if it makes you more comfortable.

## Action
1 Raise both arms toward the ceiling directly above your shoulders, palms facing each other.
2 Reach for the ceiling with one arm, stretching through the fingertips, so the shoulder blade comes off the floor, then drop the shoulder back down on to the floor.
3 Feel your upper back widening and the tension in your shoulders releasing down into the floor.
4 Repeat ten times with each arm.

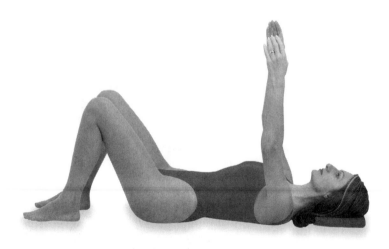

## Variation

When you are comfortable with the above, try the following variation. You will need to keep the pelvis stable, which means adding the zip up and hollow.

## Equipment

A firm flat cushion (optional).

## Starting Position

As above.

## Action

1 Breathe in, wide and full, to prepare.
2 Breathe out and zip up and hollow, keeping the pelvis still and square. Reach one hand up across to the other, toward where the ceiling meets the wall. Your shoulder blade will leave the floor. Your head should move gently with you.
3 Enjoy the stretch between the shoulder blades.
4 Breathe in and hold the stretch.
5 Breathe out and relax the shoulder back down to the floor.
6 Repeat ten times on each side, making sure that the pelvis stays quite still.

## Watchpoints

- Whatever version you are doing, maintain the distance between the ears and the shoulders.
- The shoulder blade leaves the floor, but the muscles underneath stay working.

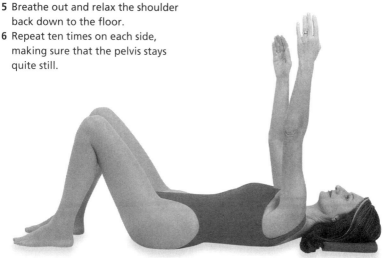

# Stage Two

# Middle Circle: Retain it!

# Spine Curls

## Aim

To learn segmental control of the spine at an intervertebral level. To have the ability to wheel the spine, vertebra by vertebra, promoting flexibility and stability throughout its length. Joseph Pilates referred to this way of moving as "using the spine like a wheel."

In a healthy back all the different segments of the spine work together to create the desired movement, each vertebra contributing to that movement a little like a bicycle chain. When one level is locked, the "chain" is upset. What often happens is that the levels above and below the locked part become overflexible to compensate for the area that will not move – you can be hypomobile (not enough movement) in one place and hypermobile (too much movement) above and/or below. This puts enormous strain on the back.

## Equipment

A firm flat cushion (optional).

## Starting Position

- Lie in the Relaxation Position, with your head on the cushion if it makes you more comfortable, your feet about eight inches from your butt, hip-width apart and parallel.
- Plant the feet firmly onto the floor and, throughout the exercise, think of the three points of the foot – the base of the big toe, the base of the little toe and the center of the heel.
- Leave your arms down by your sides, palms down.

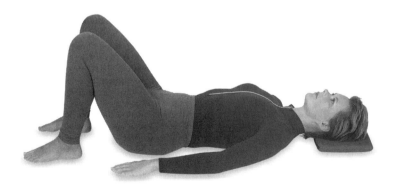

## Action

1 Breathe in, wide and full, to prepare.

2 Breathe out, zip up and hollow – stay zipped and hollowed throughout the exercise – and slowly and carefully curl just the base of your spine (the tailbone) off the floor – you will lose the neutral pelvis position.

3 Breathe in and breathe out as you lower and lengthen the spine back on to the floor.

4 Repeat, lifting a little more of the spine off the floor each time. As you lower, put each part of the spine down in sequence, bone by bone – the back of the ribs, the waist, the small of the back, the tailbone – aiming to put an imaginary two inches between each vertebra.

5 You should complete five full curls, wheeling and lengthening the spine.

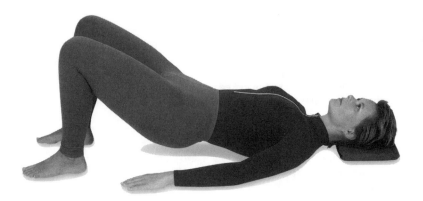

## Watchpoints

• Take care that your back does not arch and that the tailbone stays tucked under like a whippet that has just been scolded.

• Do not rush the first few curls. Really make the base of the spine move.

• There is a tendency sometimes, when there is a muscle imbalance in the torso, for one side to dominate. If you think of the spine landing like a jet on a runway, it often looks as though you are landing in a high cross wind. Try to land down the central strip of the runway – no cross winds please!

## Variations

When you feel you have mastered this exercise, you may like to try it with a cushion placed between your knees. Follow the directions above but gently squeeze the cushion as you curl.

Alternatively, while you are curled up, you may like to try the exercise taking your arms, wider than shoulder-width, behind your head to touch the floor. Only try to touch the floor if you can do so comfortably and without arching your back or flaring your ribs.

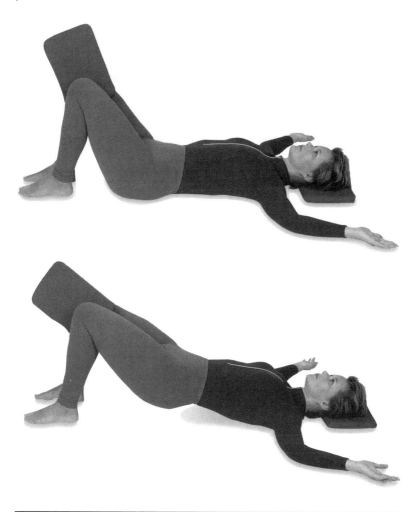

# Hip Flexor Stretch

## Aim

To lengthen the hip flexors gently.

If you sit all day, it is likely that your hip flexor muscles will shorten. If they do, this will affect the angle of your pelvis, pulling it forward (anteriorly).

## Equipment

A firm flat cushion (optional).

## Starting Position

- Lie in the Relaxation Position, with your head on the cushion if it makes you more comfortable.

## Action

1 Breathe in, wide and full, to prepare.
2 Breathe out and zip up and hollow. Keeping that sense of hollowness in the pelvis, hinge the right knee up to your chest, dropping the thigh bone down into the hip joint.
3 Breathe in as you clasp the right leg below the knee. If you have any knee problems clasp the leg under the thigh rather than below the knee so that the joint is not compressed.

4 Breathe out, zip up and hollow and stretch the left leg along the floor. Your lower back should remain in neutral. If it arches, bend the left knee back up again a little. Hold this stretch for five breaths.
5 Breathe in as you slide the leg back.
6 Breathe out and zip up and hollow as you lower the right bent knee to the floor, keeping the abdominals engaged.
7 Repeat twice on each side, keeping your shoulders relaxed and down.

## Watchpoints

- Check the position of the upper body – elbows open, breastbone soft, shoulder blades down into the back, neck released.
- Are you still in neutral?
- Slide the leg away in a line with the hip. Do not allow it to stray.

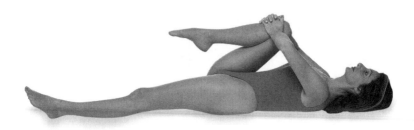

# Side Rolls

## Aim

To achieve rotation of the spine with stability. To work the obliques (the waist).

Rotation is one movement that you need to approach with caution if you have a back injury (see page 16). Always check with your medical and Pilates practitioners to see when it is safe to introduce it into your training program. At the back of the book we have given some workouts that avoid rotation (see page 197). Remember, however, that in everyday life you will be twisting and turning, so ultimately you need to be able do this safely and confidently. Some rotation is also essential to the health of the spine.

**Warning: Please seek advice if you have a disc-related injury.**

## Equipment

A firm flat cushion (optional).
A tennis ball. The purpose of the tennis ball is to help you keep good alignment of the legs and pelvis.

## Starting Position

- Lie in the Relaxation Position, with your head on the cushion if it makes you more comfortable, feet together, with the tennis ball between your knees.
- Place your arms, palms down, in a "V" shape alongside your body.
- Allow the floor to support you. Allow your body to widen and lengthen.

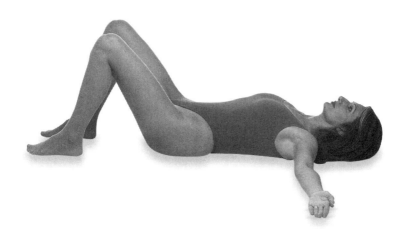

## Action

1 Breathe in, wide and full, to prepare.

2 Breathe out, zip up and hollow – stay zipped and hollowed throughout the exercise – and roll your head in one direction, your knees in the other. Only roll a little way to start with – you can go further each time as it gets more comfortable. Keep your opposite shoulder down on the floor.

3 Try to keep your knees together, the tennis ball still and the legs in line.

4 Breathe in, then breathe out, use your strong center to bring the knees back to the Starting Position. Turn your head back to the center with the movement of the knees.

5 Repeat eight times in each direction.

6 Think of rolling each part of your back off the floor in sequence and then returning the back of the ribcage, the waist, the small of your back, the butt to the floor.

## Watchpoints

• Keep the pelvis in neutral, taking care that you do not allow it to arch.

• Keep working those abdominals. Do not simply allow the weight of the legs to pull you.

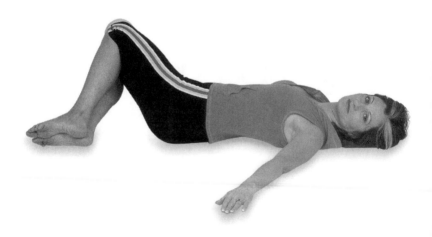

# Knee Circles with Breath

## Aim

To learn how to keep the pelvis in neutral and stable while moving the legs.

This movement stretches the lumbar spine. The gentle circular action increases the range of motion in the hip joint and encourages the lubrication of the joint with synovial fluid. It also teaches you to find neutral pelvis again and again within a movement.

**Warning: If you cannot stabilize when attempting a double knee fold, this exercise is unsuitable for you. Those with acute lower back problems should keep the pelvis neutral throughout.**

## Equipment

A firm flat cushion (optional).

## Starting Position

- Lie in the Relaxation Position with your head on the cushion if it makes you more comfortable.

- Zip up and hollow and bring your knees up and hip-width apart toward your chest, one at a time.
- Cradle each knee in a relaxed hand and allow the legs to hang, but take care that this does not arch your lower back.
- Your elbows stay open and the shoulders relaxed.

## Action

1 Breathe in, wide and full, to prepare.
2 Breathe out, zip up and hollow and stay zipped and hollowed throughout the exercise.
3 The aim is to circle the knees as if you are stirring the leg in the hip joint, so breathe in as you draw both knees further into the chest. The pelvis will tilt posteriorly at this point.
4 Breathe out as you part the knees and let them circle back to the starting position. At this point the pelvis will rock back into the neutral position.
5 Repeat eight times.

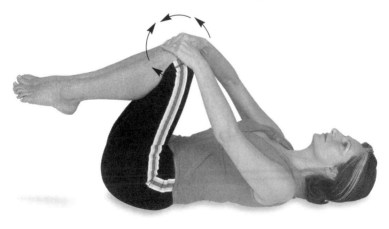

### Variation

This movement can also be reversed.

1 Start with both knees together and pulled into the chest, the pelvis tilted posteriorly.
2 Breathe out as both legs circle away from the body (knees together). The pelvis rocks back into neutral and you stabilize at this point.
3 Breathe in as you part the knees and pull them gently toward your chest.

### Watchpoints

- Watch out for uneven circles, which indicate that you may have less flexibility in one hip. If this is the case, focus on releasing that hip.
- Keep the upper body relaxed and open at all times. Imagine that the legs are light.
- Make sure you regain the neutral pelvis and keep a strong center.

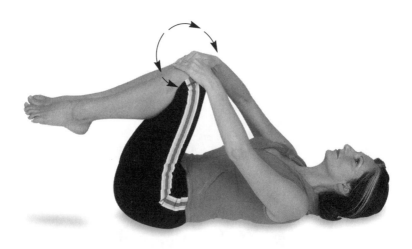

# Windmill Arms

## Aim
To improve coordination, mobilize the shoulder girdle and improve scapular stabilizing skills.

## Equipment
A firm flat cushion (optional).

## Starting Position
- Lie in the Relaxation Position, with your head on the cushion if it makes you more comfortable and with your pelvis in neutral.
- Both arms should be pointing up to the ceiling, directly above your shoulder joints. Long fingers, palms facing toward your feet, elbows soft.

## Action
1 Breathe in, wide and full, to prepare.
2 Breathe out, zip up and hollow, and let the right arm move in an arc behind you on to the floor as far as is comfortable, while, at the same time, the left arm moves toward the hip. This is the same movement as for the Starfish.
3 The palm of the right hand should face the ceiling, the left palm the floor.
4 Breathe in and rotate the arms slowly along the mat in opposite directions, like a windmill, so that the arms change places. You end up with the left hand (palm facing up) behind you and the right hand (palm facing down) next to your hip.

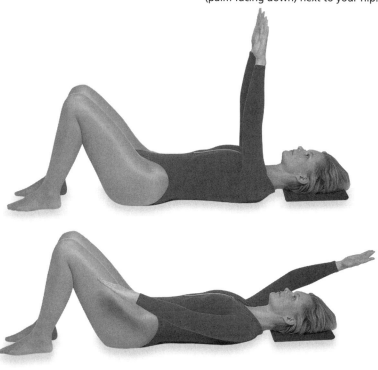

**5** Breathe out to lift both arms off the mat and return to the Starting Position.

**6** Repeat the same movement five times.

### *Advanced Version*
Reverse the movement after each time – very challenging for the brain!

### Watchpoints
- Maintain neutral spine and pelvis throughout.
- Keep your shoulders down and do not force the arms all the way to the mat. Work within your comfortable range of movement.

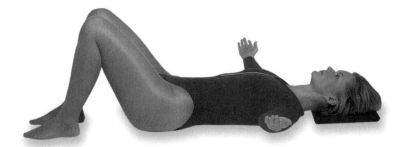

# Walking on the Spot plus Calf Stretch

## Aim

To warm up the legs, mobilize the ankle joints, reaffirm good leg alignment and stretch the calves gently. It also starts to get the circulation going.

A simple exercise that can be done anywhere, it is deceptively hard to do well. It is particularly useful before, during and after flying because it works the calf pump, which helps prevent deep-vein thrombosis. The key to doing this exercise properly is to keep good body alignment throughout. You have three main body weights – your head, your ribcage and your pelvis. Try to keep them balanced centrally on top of each other. When you bend your knees in this exercise they should bend directly over the second toes. You may have to check this occasionally during the exercise.

## Starting Position

- Stand correctly (see page 66).
- Your feet should be hip-width apart.

## Action

1 Breathing normally, come up on to the balls of your feet, making sure that your body does not pitch forward.
2 Drop your left heel back down, your right knee bending over your foot as you do so.
3 Swap legs so that you are, in effect, walking on the spot. The idea is to keep lengthening upward while your weight stays centered, your pelvis level and your waist long.

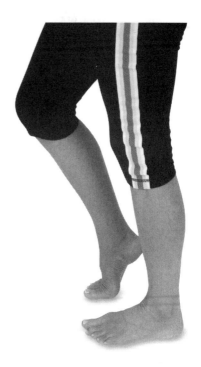

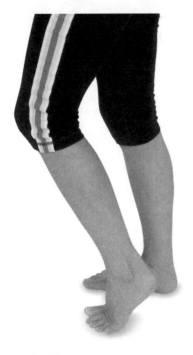 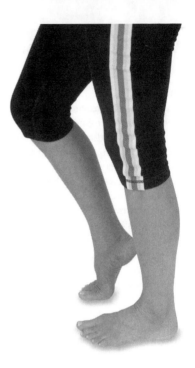

### *Moving On*

When you get the hang of this, you can add an extra movement by bending the knee of the leg that is "flat" on the floor. This should give you a gentle stretch in the calf.

Make sure the knee bends directly over the second toe.

### Watchpoints

- Check that when you bend your knee, it bends over the center of the foot – over the second toe, to be precise.
- Try not to lean forward.
- Do not collapse.
- Try not to wiggle your hips around. Your pelvis stays level and neutral throughout.

# Arm Circles against the Wall

## Aim

To mobilize the shoulder girdle and to improve scapular stabilizing skills.

The idea of this exercise is for the hands to move along the wall while keeping the body well aligned. However, it is pointless to force the arms back, especially since this will probably result in you arching your back and flaring your ribcage. Work within your comfort range of movement, paying close attention to good technique.

## Action

1 Breathe in, wide and full, to prepare.
2 Breathe out, zip up and hollow – stay zipped and hollowed throughout the exercise – and reach your arms out in front of you, palms down, and then lift them above your head. Lengthen through your fingers and keep your shoulder blades drawing down into your back.

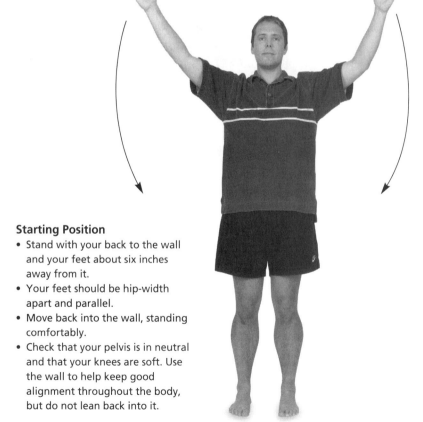

## Starting Position

- Stand with your back to the wall and your feet about six inches away from it.
- Your feet should be hip-width apart and parallel.
- Move back into the wall, standing comfortably.
- Check that your pelvis is in neutral and that your knees are soft. Use the wall to help keep good alignment throughout the body, but do not lean back into it.

**3** As you breathe out reach your arms out to the sides, palms facing forward, and lengthen your arms down to the sides of your body. Repeat six times. Then reverse the circle, exhaling as the arms lift up and inhaling as the arms move down.

**Watchpoints**

- Maintain neutral pelvis and neutral spine throughout and do not allow the upper back to arch away from the wall.
- Do not allow the ribs to flare. Move with the breath.
- Keep the shoulder blades wide and down the back, but do allow for mobility. No gripping! Stay relaxed.
- Keep the neck long and released.
- Watch the alignment of the hands and wrists.
- Keep the elbows soft.

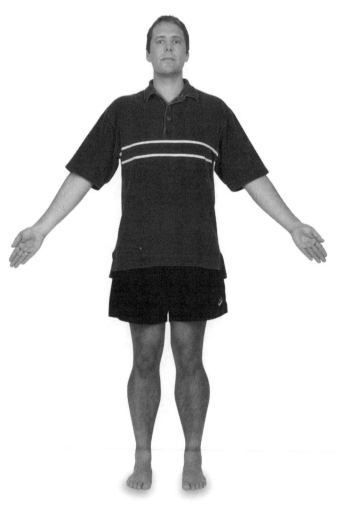

# Version Two (Arm Circles: Free Standing)

Once arm circles can be performed against the wall while core stability is maintained and you have good shoulder mobility, move away from the wall and perform the exercise free-standing.

Follow all the directions above.

**Watchpoints**
- Maintain zip up and hollow throughout.
- Keep your weight evenly balanced on both feet.
- Do not allow the range of arm movement to go too far – you must maintain the connection with the shoulder blades.
- Keep checking that your back is not arching.

# Side Reach against the Wall

## Aim
To stretch the sides of the trunk and learn good lateral flexion of the spine.

## Starting Position
- Stand with your back against a wall, your feet a few inches away from it. Have your feet just wider than shoulder-width apart and parallel.
- Lean back into the wall and notice where your body touches it. Do not tip your head back to touch the wall, it should be balanced on top of the spine.
- Check that your pelvis is in neutral.
- Your hands are resting on the outside of your thighs.

**NOTE** Keep the non-working arm in contact with the outside of the thigh throughout the stretch.

## Action
1 Breathe in, wide and full, to prepare and lengthen through the spine.
2 Breathe out, zip up and hollow – stay zipped and hollowed throughout the exercise – and slowly raise one arm up to the side and above your head, trying to keep the arm in contact with the wall (do not force it).
3 Breathe in wide, and just check that your shoulder blade is still connected down into your back and that there is a large gap between your ears and your shoulders. Lengthen up through the top of your head.
4 Breathe out, and lift up out of your waist to reach toward the top corner of the room. Keep your head in a line with your spine (face forward still) and do not move away from the wall.
5 Breathe in and slowly return to the center.
6 Breathe out and lower the arm along the wall.
7 Repeat five times to each side.

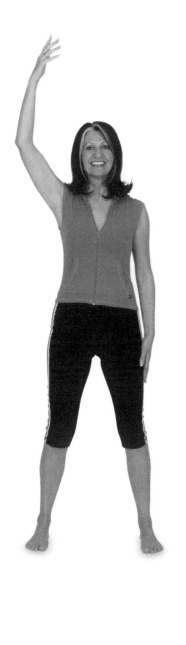

### Watchpoints
- Keep noting where your body is touching the wall.
- Keep your pelvis central and do not allow it to shift to one side.
- Keep both feet firmly on the floor.

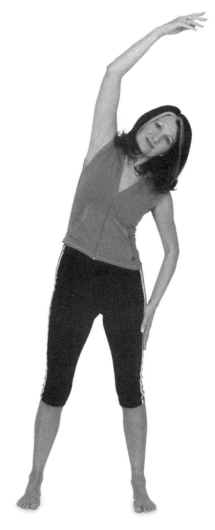

# Dumb Waiter on the Wall

### Aim
To become aware of the shoulder
blades and how they move on the
ribcage. To open the chest and
strengthen the muscles between the
shoulder blades.

### Starting Position
- Stand with your back against a wall,
  feet hip-width apart, parallel and
  approximately eight inches away
  from the wall.
- Lean back into the wall, checking
  that your pelvis is in neutral. Do not
  push your head on to the wall; allow
  it to balance on top of the spine.
- Hold both arms out in front of you
  as if holding an imaginary tray of
  hors d'oeuvres.
- Your palms face upward, elbows
  stay close to your trunk.

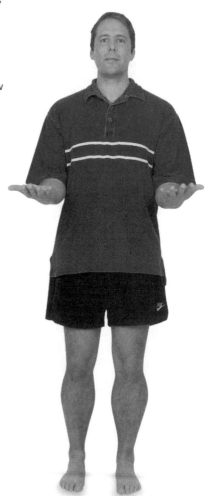

## Action

1 Breathe in, wide and full, to prepare and lengthen through the spine.
2 Breathe out, zip up and hollow and stay zipped and hollowed throughout the exercise.
3 Breathe in and, keeping your elbows still and close to your torso, take your forearms to the side as far as you can go. The forearms stay parallel to the floor, the shoulder blades stay down and the chest opens.
4 Breathe out and return to the Starting Position.
5 Repeat five to ten times.

## Watchpoints

• The upper back should not arch off the wall as you take the arms back.
• Feel the shoulder blades moving equally on the wall.
• Keep your weight evenly balanced on both feet.

# Knee Swings

## Aim

To learn pelvic stability and to stretch the hip rotator muscles.

This is a lovely exercise for promoting hip mobility. As you practice it more, you will find you develop a much greater range of movement at the hip.

## Equipment

A small cushion (optional).

## Starting Position

- Lie on your front with your body in a straight line and your forehead resting on your folded hands. If you need to, place a small cushion underneath your stomach.
- Check that your upper body is completely relaxed and that your neck is lengthened and released.
- Bend one knee up to 90°.

## Action

1 Breathe in, wide and full, to prepare and lengthen through the body.
2 Breathe out, zip up and hollow – stay zipped and hollowed throughout the exercise – and allow the bent leg to fall outward, keeping the knee and pelvis quite still.
3 Breathe in and return the bent leg to the center of the sweep.
4 Breathe out and bring the leg inward, keeping the leg on the floor and pelvis still.
5 Breathe in and recover.
6 Repeat ten times with each leg.

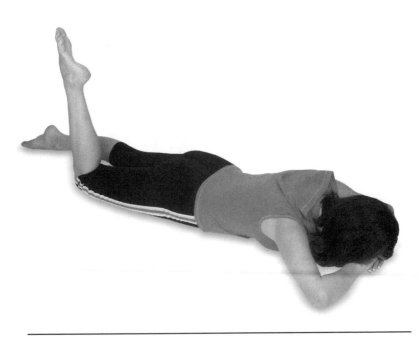

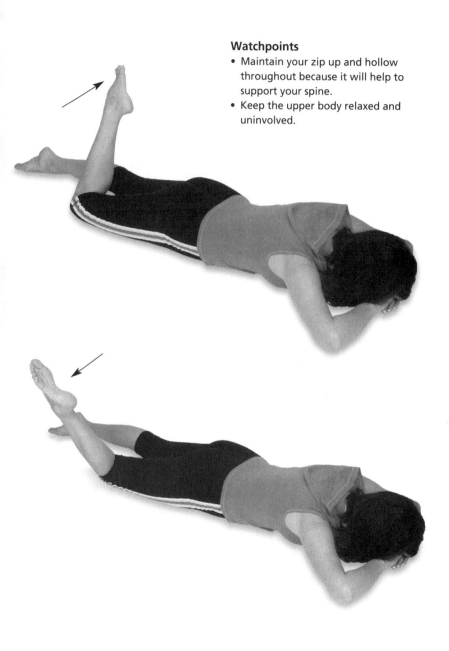

### Watchpoints

- Maintain your zip up and hollow throughout because it will help to support your spine.
- Keep the upper body relaxed and uninvolved.

# The Oyster

## Aim

To strengthen the gluteus medius, which is a very important muscle for stabilizing the pelvis. It is also a very good exercise if you have knee problems.

## Equipment

A firm flat cushion.

## Starting Position

- Lie in a straight line on your side.
- Have your underneath arm stretched out above your head in a line with your body, and place the cushion between your ear and arm so that your neck is in a line with your spine.
- Bend your knees, keeping your feet in a line with your butt (see photo).

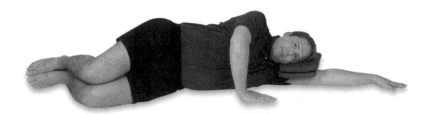

## Action

1 Breathe in, wide and full, to prepare.
2 Breathe out, zip up and hollow – stay zipped and hollowed throughout the exercise – and slowly rotate your top leg, opening the knee and keeping the feet together on top of each other. The action initiates in the butt.
3 Make sure that as you do so you do not lose your neutral pelvis or spine; keep lengthening through the body.
4 Breathe in and hold.
5 Breathe out and close.
6 Repeat ten times on each side.

## Watchpoints

- Do not allow your waist to sink into the floor, keep it long.
- Do not allow your upper body to fall forward.
- Maintain a neutral pelvis throughout.

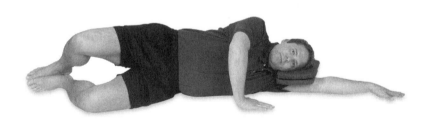

# The Big Squeeze

## Aim
To work the muscles of the lower abdomen, pelvic floor, the butt and the inner thighs (adductors) while keeping the upper body relaxed.

## Equipment
A small cushion.

## Starting Position
- Lie on your front.
- Place, or get a close friend to place, a small cushion between the tops of your thighs.
- Rest your forehead on your folded hands. Your shoulders are open and relaxed.
- Have your toes together and your heels apart.

## Action
1 Breathe in, wide and full, to prepare and lengthen through the spine.
2 Breathe out, zip up and hollow the lower abdominals toward the spine as if there were a fragile egg under your stomach that you do not want to crush.

3 Tighten the butt, squeeze the inner thighs and the cushion, and bring the heels together. Hold for a count of five.
4 Keep breathing normally and keep checking that you are only working from the waist down. Then release.
5 Keep your feet on the floor.
6 Repeat the Big Squeeze five times.

## Watchpoints
- Keep your neck and jaw relaxed as you squeeze.
- Feel the full length of your body from the top of your head to the tips of your toes.
- As you squeeze, think of lengthening the base of the spine.

### Moving On
Try engaging the muscles in this order: pelvic floor, lower abdominals, butt, inner thigh. Then release in reverse order – fun!

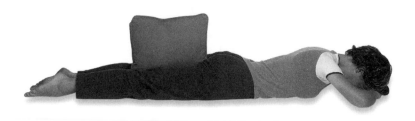

# The Star

We have added an extra stage (taking the leg to the side) to this classic Pilates exercise.

## Aim

To learn how to work from a strong stable center. To work the deep gluteal muscles and the upper back muscles. To learn how to extend the leg safely.

## Stage One

### Equipment

A small flat cushion (optional).

### Starting Position

- Lie on your front with your feet hip-width apart and turned out from the hips. If you are uncomfortable lying on your stomach, place a small flat cushion under your abdomen to tilt the pelvis and start gently. If you have a history of sciatica, leave the legs parallel.
- Rest your forehead on your folded arms.

### Action

1 Breathe in, wide and full, to prepare, and lengthen through the spine.

2 Breathe out, zip up and hollow – stay zipped and hollowed throughout the exercise – and first lengthen then raise the left leg, lifting it no more than two inches off the ground. Lengthen away from a strong center. Do not twist the pelvis; both hip joints should stay on the floor.
3 Try to keep your shoulders relaxed and a sense of width in your upper body.
4 Breathe in and relax.
5 Repeat five times with each leg.

### Watchpoints

- Keep the lower abdominals supporting your lower back.
- Think of creating space around the hip joint as you lengthen the leg away.
- Be careful to keep both hips on the floor – you are only lifting the leg.
- Don't let the pelvis roll or twist, keep it square.
- Keep your neck long and relaxed; the head stays down on the floor throughout the exercise.
- Everyone lifts the legs too high to begin with; aim to lift just a few inches.

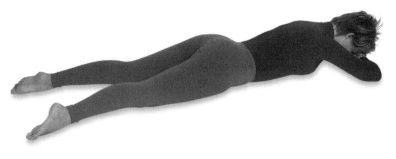

# Stage Two

## Equipment and Starting Position
Same as Stage One.

## Action
1 Breathe in, wide and full, to prepare.
2 Breathe out, zip up and hollow – stay zipped and hollowed throughout the exercise – and slide one leg to the side. Only take the leg as far as you can keep the pelvis still. Do not allow one side of your trunk to shorten.
3 Breathe in and return the leg to the starting position.
4 Repeat five times on each side.

## Watchpoints
- Keep your upper body relaxed and uninvolved.
- Stay zipped and hollowed so that your low back is supported.
- Check that you do not allow the hip to "hitch up" as the leg moves to the side.
- Keep lengthening through the leg.

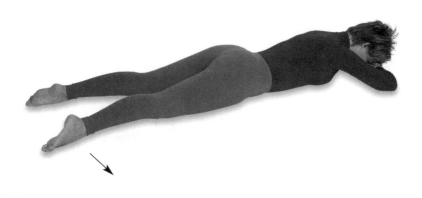

# Stage Three: The Full Star

## Equipment
A small very flat cushion or a towel (optional).

## Starting Position
- Take your arms out just wider than shoulder width so that you look like a star, but remember to leave your shoulder blades set down in your back.
- You may like to place a small, very flat cushion or folded towel under your forehead. The cushion should not alter the angle of your neck.

## Action
1 Breathe in, wide and full, to prepare and lengthen through the spine.
2 Breathe out, zip up and hollow – stay zipped and hollowed throughout the exercise – and first lengthen, then raise, the opposite arm and leg no more than two inches off the ground. Lengthen away from a strong center. Do not twist in the pelvis; both hip joints stay on the floor.

3 Try to keep a sense of width in your upper body.
4 Breathe in and relax.
5 Repeat five times each side.

## Watchpoints
- Do not overreach or overlift the arms. Keep the elbows slightly bent and keep them wide.
- Keep your neck long and relaxed; the head stays down on the floor throughout the exercise.

When you have finished the Star come on to all fours into the Rest Position.

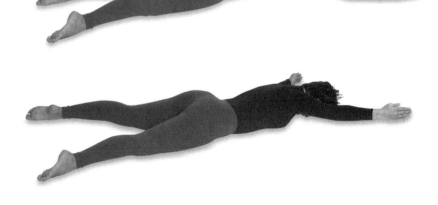

# The Rest Position: Two Versions

We have given you two versions of this exercise. The first focuses on the movement back from four-point kneeling on to your heels. This helps to teach you good alignment. The second version adds an inner-thigh stretch. If you find this position compresses your knees too much, place a pillow behind the knees.

**Warning: Avoid sitting back on your heels if you have knee problems.**

## Version One (Moving Back)

### Aim
To lengthen and stretch out your sacral, lumbar, middle and upper spine.

### Equipment
A plump cushion (optional).

### Starting Position
- Ideally you should do this exercise alongside a mirror so that you can check your spinal and pelvic alignment as you move back.
- Come on to all fours, your hands directly beneath your shoulders, fingers facing forward.
- Your knees are in a line with your hips, your feet are together.

- Your neck should be lengthened and, unless you are looking in the mirror, you should be looking straight down.
- Check that your spine has maintained its natural curves and that your pelvis is in neutral.
- The back should look neither too flat nor overly dipped.

### Action
1 Breathe in, wide and full, to prepare and lengthen through the spine.
2 Breathe out, zip up and hollow – stay zipped and hollowed throughout the exercise – and slowly start to move your butt backward. Breathe normally as you inch back. The idea is to keep the natural curve in the back and not allow it to flatten. It helps to think of sticking your butt out or to think of keeping a pool of water in the small of your back.
3 Go as far back as you can. Hopefully, you should be able to rest your butt on your heels. If you are not that flexible, place a plump cushion on your heels for your butt to rest on.
4 Once in this position, take the opportunity to breathe deeply into your back and sides.
5 To come out of this position see below.

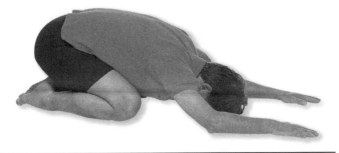

# Version Two (Inner-thigh Stretch)

## Aim

To lengthen and stretch out your sacral, lumbar, middle and upper spine. To stretch your inner thighs (adductors). To learn to control your breathing in a relaxed position, to sense the filling and emptying of the lungs. To make maximum use of the lungs, taking the breath into the back.

**Warning: Avoid sitting back on your heels if you have knee problems. We do not recommend this version for anyone with back injuries.**

## Equipment and Starting Position

Same as Version One.

## Action

1 Do steps 1 and 2 from Version One until you reach a kneeling position, then bring your feet together, your knees staying apart. Slowly move your butt back toward your feet.
2 Do not raise your head or hands Rest your butt on your heels – not between them; the back is rounded.

3 Rest and relax into this position, leave the arms extended to give you a maximum stretch. Feel the expansion of the back of your ribcage as you breathe deeply into it.
4 The further apart the knees are, the more of a stretch you will feel in your inner thighs (adductors), the more you can think of your chest sinking down into the floor.
5 Alternatively, you may have the knees together, which will stretch the lumbar spine.
6 Take ten breaths in this position.

## To come out of the Rest Position

- As you breathe out, zip up and hollow and slowly unfurl.
- Think of dropping your tailbone down and bringing your pubic bone forward.
- Rebuild your spine vertebra by vertebra until you are upright. As you do so, think of keeping your head and shoulders relaxed and open.

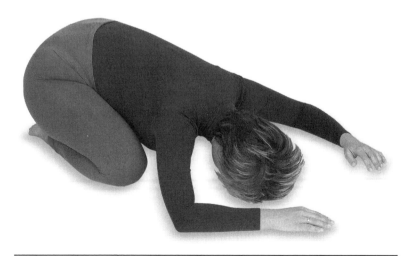

# Curl Ups

## Aim

To strengthen the abdominals, engaging them in the correct order with the trunk in perfect alignment. To achieve a flat stomach – well, we all want one!

**Warning: Avoid this exercise if you have neck problems.**

## Equipment

A firm flat cushion (optional).

## Starting Position

- Lie in the Relaxation Position, with your head on the cushion if it makes you more comfortable.
- Place one hand behind your head, the other on your lower abdomen. This is to check that your stomach does not pop up.
- Your pelvis is in its neutral position.

## Action

1 Gently release your neck by rolling the head slowly from side to side.
2 Breathe in, wide and full, to prepare.
3 Breathe out, zip up and hollow and stay zipped and hollowed throughout the exercise.
4 Soften your breastbone, tuck your chin in a little and curl up, breaking from the breastbone. Think of your ribcage funneling down toward your waist.

5 Your stomach must not pop up. Keep the length and width in the front of the pelvis and the tailbone down on the floor lengthening away. Do not tuck the pelvis or pull on the neck.
6 Breathe in and slowly curl back down.
7 Repeat ten times (change hands after five).

## Watchpoints

- Try not to grip around the hips.
- Stay in neutral, tailbone down on the floor and lengthening away.
- The front of the body keeps its length. A useful image is of a strip of sticky tape along the front of the body that should not wrinkle!

### Moving On

Once you are confident that your pelvis remains in neutral and your lower abdominals do not pop up, you should place both hands behind your head. Keep your elbows open so they are just in your line of vision. Do not pull on your head or neck but, rather, allow the head to rest in your hands.

Follow the directions above.

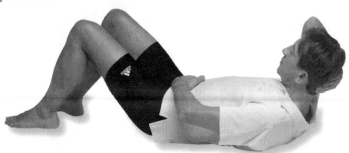

# Oblique Curl Ups

## Aim
To work the oblique muscles.

**Warning: Avoid this exercise if you have neck problems.**

## Equipment and Starting Position
As for the previous exercise, only place both hands behind your head, the elbows staying open and still within your line of vision.

## Action
1 Breathe in, wide and full, to prepare.
2 Breathe out, zip up and hollow – stay zipped and hollowed throughout the exercise – and bring your left shoulder across toward your right knee. The elbow stays back, it is the shoulder that moves forward.
3 Your stomach must stay hollow, the pelvis stable.
4 Breathe in and lower.
5 Repeat five times on each side.

## Watchpoints
- As for Curl Ups, make sure that the pelvis stays square and stable.
- Keep the upper body open
- Keep the neck released.

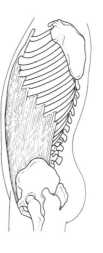 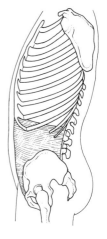

External oblique        Internal oblique

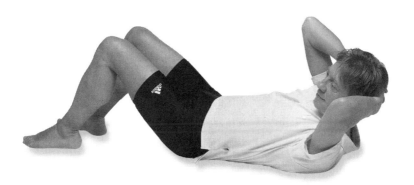

# Hamstring Stretch

## Aim

To stretch the hamstrings while keeping the torso stable, the back anchored and without creating any tension elsewhere in the body.

In addition to gentle hamstring stretches, you will also need to strengthen the gluteals through exercises such as the Oyster on page 112.

**Warning: If you suffer from sciatica or disc-related problems, please seek advice before trying this exercise.**

## Equipment

One or two small flat cushions (optional).
A scarf or stretch band.

## Starting Position

- Lie in the Relaxation Position, with your head on the cushion if it makes you more comfortable
- Bend one knee upward toward your chest.
- Holding the scarf from underneath, with your palms toward you, place it over the sole of one foot.
- Check that you have returned to neutral.

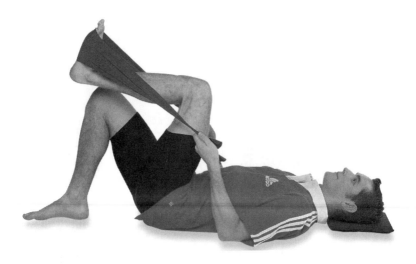

## Action

1 Breathe in, wide and full, to prepare.
2 Breathe out, zip up and hollow – stay zipped and hollowed throughout the exercise – and slowly straighten the leg into the air. Keep the foot relaxed; think of lengthening through the heel. Make sure that the leg stays parallel, your kneecap facing you in a line with your hip. Keep your tailbone down on the floor, the pelvis staying neutral north and south, west and east.
3 Breathing normally now, hold the stretch for a count of about thirty seconds or until you feel the muscles release.
4 Relax the leg by bending it again gently.
5 Repeat five times on each leg.

## Watchpoints

• Don't allow the pelvis to twist as you straighten the leg.
• Keep your tailbone down as you stretch the leg.
• Check your neck. Often the neck shortens and arches back as the hamstrings are stretched. If this happens, place another small flat firm cushion under your head to keep the neck long.
• Think of softening the neck and breastbone and of opening the elbows. Hold the scarf so that, if possible, your elbows stay down on the floor.
• Check that your shoulder blades stay down into your back.
• Don't strain – ease the leg out, gently stretching it within your limits.

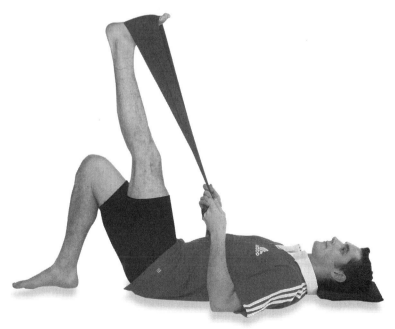

# Adductor Openings

### Aim

To stretch the inner thighs (adductors) gently, with the pelvis in neutral.

The muscles of the inner thigh – the adductors

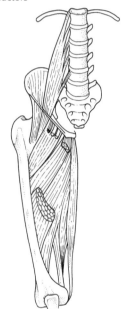

### Equipment

A firm flat cushion (optional).

### Starting Position

- Lie in the Relaxation Position, with your head on the cushion if it makes you more comfortable.

### Action

1 Breathe in, wide and full, to prepare.
2 Breathe out, zip up and hollow and bring one knee at a time on to your chest.
3 Breathing normally now, place one hand under each knee and allow the legs to open slowly until you can feel the stretch.
4 This will stretch your inner thighs (adductors). Hold this position for two minutes or until you feel the muscle release. Do not allow your back to arch.
5 After two minutes, slowly close the legs, zip up and hollow, and return your feet one at a time to the floor.

### Watchpoint

- Stay in neutral.

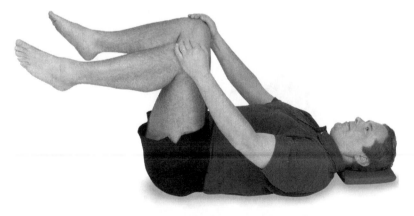

# Wide Leg Stretch against the Wall

A more adventurous stretch for the inner thighs (adductors), this is also a lovely position to relax in. With the legs elevated, the calf pump, which returns blood to the heart, has to work harder, improving your circulation and your lymphatic drainage, thus helping to prevent varicose veins, swelling in the legs and the build-up of toxins.

## Equipment
A small flat cushion.

## Starting Position and Action
- Get into the position shown in the photograph – it is easiest to approach the wall sideways and shuffle up as close to it as you can, then slowly swing your legs up the wall.

- You must still be comfortable.
- Rest your head on a flat cushion.
- Check that you are square on to the wall.
- You may put your hands under your butt if it helps, and you should certainly do this if you have back problems. If your hamstrings are tight, then come back from the wall a little.
- Move your legs apart into a wide stretch.
- Your tailbone must stay down on the floor or you lose neutral.

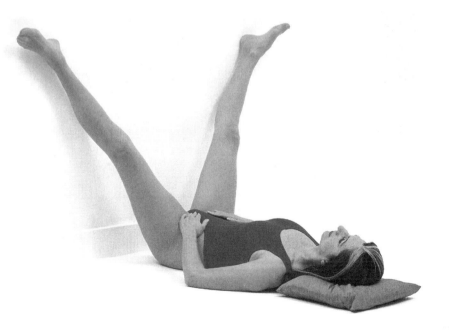

# Chicken Wings on the Wall

## Aim

To strengthen the scapular stabilizers and stretch the upper chest. Standing against the wall also strengthens your thigh muscles.

## Equipment

A scarf, a stretch band or a light stick from the garden.

## Starting Position

- Stand with your back against a wall with your feet hip-width apart, parallel, and approximately eight inches away from the wall.
- Lean back into the wall, checking that your pelvis is in neutral. Your head will probably be away from the wall; do not force it back, just allow it to balance on top of the spine.
- Hold the band or stick in front of you with your arms a little more than shoulder-width apart.
- Maintain a soft curve in the arms.

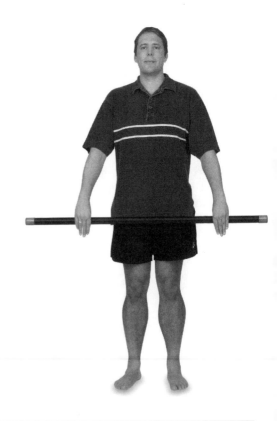

## Action

1 Breathe in, wide and full, to lengthen the spine.
2 Breathe out, zip up and hollow and stay zipped and hollowed throughout the exercise.
3 Breathe in and slowly raise both arms up as far as you can go without arching your back.
4 Breathe out and bend both elbows. The band will go toward the top of your head or forehead, depending on your flexibility. The shoulder blades are gliding down the back.

5 Breathe in and almost straighten the elbows, keeping the shoulder blades down into the back.
6 Breathe out and lower the arms to the Starting Position.
7 Repeat up to ten times.

## Watchpoints

- Keep your upper shoulders relaxed when you raise your arms.
- Do not force your arms back to touch the wall if it means you are arching your ribs.
- Remember to keep your arms soft, with your elbows bent. Move both arms at the same time. (This is easier to check if you are working with a stick).

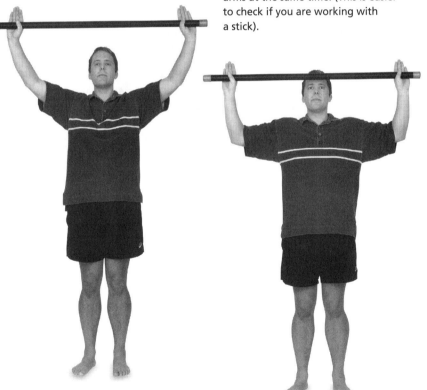

# Floating Arms against the Wall

## Aim

To strengthen the muscles around the shoulders. To learn good alignment and upper-body use.

This exercise is a natural progression from Floating Arms (page 79) and the Starfish (page 82). Remember to focus on the alignment of the rest of your body.

## Starting Position

- Stand with your back to the wall and your feet about three inches away from it.
- Notice which parts of your body are touching the wall; find your neutral pelvis position.
- Do not be tempted to tip your head back to the wall, and keep lengthening up through the top of your head.

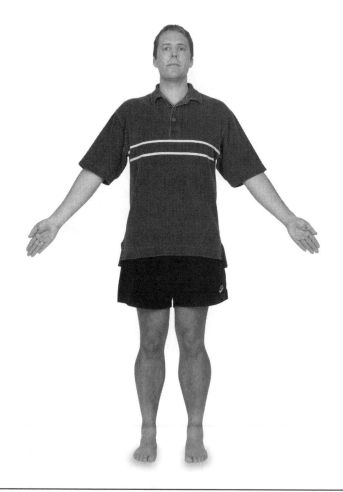

## Action

1 Breathe in, wide and full, to prepare.

2 Breathe out, zip up and hollow – stay zipped and hollowed throughout the exercise – and slowly raise your arms, sliding your shoulder blades down into your back. Keep your arms fairly straight, but your elbows soft. Do not force the arms back or allow your back to arch at all.

3 Breathe in, wide and full, and hold this position.

4 Breathe out and slowly lower your arms.

5 Repeat five times.

## Watchpoints

• Keep your neutral pelvis position throughout.

• Keep your upper body soft and open.

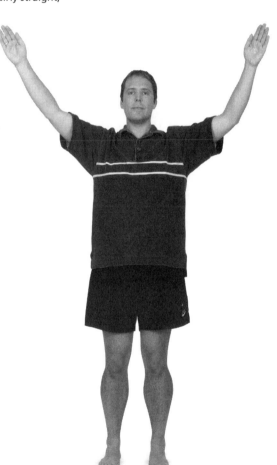

# Sitting Waist Twists

### Aim
To learn safe rotation of the spine, adding length and stability.

**Warning: Since this exercise involves rotation of the spine, please consult your medical practitioner if you have a disc-related injury.**

### Equipment
A strong pole about five feet in length. A thick bamboo pole is ideal because it retains some flexibility. A straight-backed chair.

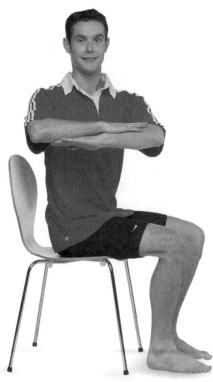

### Starting Position
- Sit on a chair, your feet firmly planted, hip-width apart, on the floor.
- If you can, place the pole across your shoulders. If this is not comfortable, fold your arms in front of you, in line with your chest.
- Keep your shoulders down and your neck soft.

### Action
1 Breathe in and lengthen up through your spine.
2 Breathe out, zip up and hollow – stay zipped and hollowed throughout the exercise – and turn to the right as far as you can while keeping your pelvis square and facing forward. Your arms stay at chest height.
3 Breathe in to lengthen up, and return to the front.
4 Repeat five times to each side. Remember to keep lengthening up.

### Watchpoints
- Do not allow the shoulders to creep up around the ears. Keep the shoulder blades down into the back.
- Try to keep the weight evenly balanced on both buttcheeks and on both feet.
- Do not turn the head too far. It should move naturally, balanced on top of the spine.
- Try not to tilt forward with one shoulder; stay central.

# Standing Waist Twists

### Aim
Same as Sitting Waist Twists.

### Equipment
A strong pole about five feet in length. A thick bamboo pole is ideal because it retains some flexibility.

### Starting Position
- Stand tall, remembering all the directions given on page 66.
- Place the pole across your shoulders, taking your arms around and under with your hands resting on the pole. If this is too uncomfortable, hold your arms out to the side. If they tire, lower them as necessary.

### Action
1 Breathe in as you lengthen up through the spine.
2 Breathe out, zip up and hollow – stay zipped and hollowed throughout the exercise – and, keeping your pelvis square and facing forward, gently turn your upper body around as far as is comfortable. Your head turns with your body
3 Only turn as far as you can keep your pelvis square and still.
4 Breathe in as you return to center.
5 Repeat up to ten times to each side.

### Watchpoints
- Same as for the previous exercise, but you will have to work harder and pay close attention to keeping the correct pelvic alignment.
- If you find your pelvis moving, stand in front of a table or the back of a chair with your thighs just touching it – this gives you an idea of when you twist your pelvis.

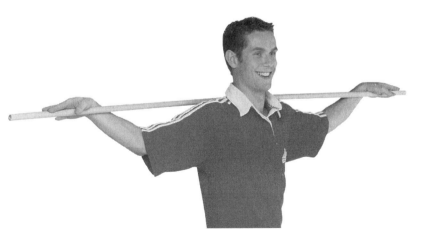

# Standing on One Leg

## Aim

To learn to balance the core areas of the trunk, pelvis and scapulae, working from a strong center. To work the muscles of the ankles and feet. To work each leg individually. To learn how to achieve pelvic stability, working the deep posterior fibers of gluteus medius.

We all tend to favor one leg, which can, as a result, grow stronger than its partner. This can have repercussions throughout the body. Exercises that require you to stand on one leg help to strengthen the weaker leg. They also work on the deep butt muscle, gluteus medius, which, if weak, can cause the opposite quadratus lumborum, a deep muscle situated on each side of the trunk, to become too strong.

It is very useful to do this exercise in front of a mirror so you can check that your pelvis stays level.

If you find yourself wobbling too much, practice by holding on to the back of a chair.

## Starting Position

- Stand in a balanced way, reminding yourself of all the directions given on page 66.

## Action

1 Breathe in and lengthen up through the spine.
2 Breathe out, zip up and hollow and take the weight on to one leg, keeping the pelvis completely level. Do not tip to one side. Lift the other leg a little way off the floor. Keep lengthening up, maintaining a long waist on both sides.
3 Find your balance and breathe normally for a few breaths before returning the foot to the floor.
4 Repeat five times on each leg.

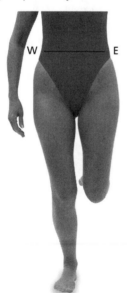

keep the pelvis level

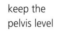

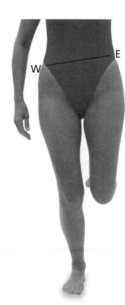

do not allow it to tilt

### Variation One

This variation demonstrates clearly how much we rely on our visual sense to stay balanced. Without the visual messages to the brain, it has to rely on all the other senses.

Repeat the instructions for Standing on One Leg but this time try closing your eyes.

### Watchpoints

- Try not to sink into the hip of the leg you are standing on.
- Keep lengthening your waist on both sides.
- Do not shift your weight to one side; stay centered.
- The pelvis must stay level.

### Variation Two

- Follow the instructions for Standing on One Leg but this time, instead of bending the leg, slide it forward along the floor, then turn the leg out from the hip, keeping the pelvis level and still.
- Make sure that the action originates from the hip and not the knee. Think of the whole leg spiraling out from the hip.
- Bring the leg back into parallel and slide it back.
- Repeat five times on each side.

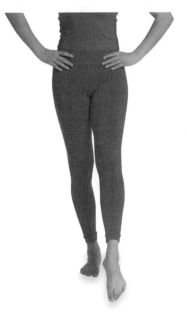

### Watchpoints

- Remember how you turned the leg out in the Pelvic Stability Exercises (page 73) and try to achieve the same – the movement happens in the hip joint.

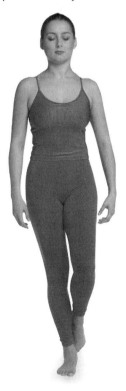

# Table Top: Stages One and Two

## Aim

To learn how to keep your center stabilized while moving the limbs, maintaining neutral and keeping the length in the trunk. To learn balance and control. To learn pelvic stability and to work the deep gluteals.

The key to this exercise is to keep your girdle of strength supporting the spine and keeping both sides of the waist long, the pelvis neutral and level. No tension should creep into the upper body.

A complementary exercise would be Standing on One Leg, page 132.

## Stage One

### Starting Position for Stages One and Two

- Kneel on all fours, your hands directly beneath your shoulders, fingertips forward and weight evenly balanced on the whole hand, not just the heels of the hands.

- Your knees should be beneath your hips.
- Check that your pelvis is neutral and the natural curve in your back maintained – think of a pool of water resting in the small of your back.

## Action

1 Breathe in, wide and full, to prepare, as you lengthen the spine from the top of your head to your tailbone.
2 Breathe out, zip up and hollow – stay zipped and hollowed throughout the exercise – and slide the right leg away from you, straightening it along the floor.
3 Breathe in and slowly return the leg.
4 Repeat five times with each leg.

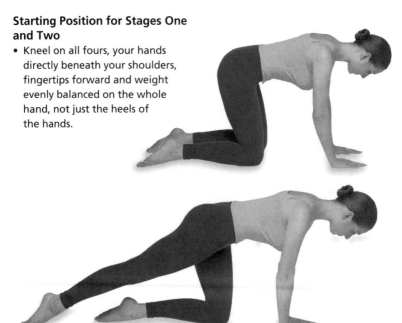

## Stage Two

When you have mastered the above –
always keeping your center stable –
you may try the next stage.

### Action

1 Follow steps 1–2 above.
2 After lengthening the leg along the
  floor, breathe in then out as you
  slowly lift the leg to hip-height, but
  no higher!
3 The pelvis must stay absolutely level.
  Do not allow the low back to over-
  dip or tilt.
4 Repeat five times with each leg.

### Watchpoints

- Try to keep the weight evenly
  balanced on both hands.
- Keep your shoulder blades down
  into your back, your elbows open
  and your neck long.
- Keep lengthening through the
  straightened leg.
- Keep both sides of the waist long.
- If your wrists ache, stop for a
  moment, then carry on. They will
  eventually become stronger.

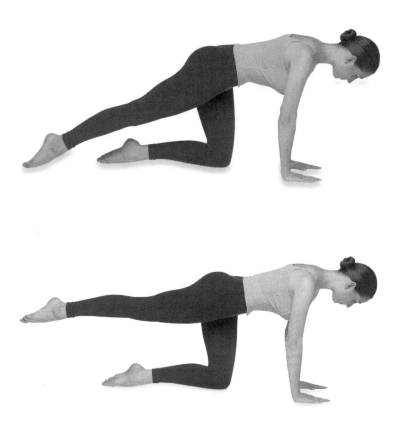

# The Diamond Press

## Aim

To develop awareness of the scapulae moving on the ribcage. To work the muscles that stabilize the shoulder blades, especially lower trapezius. To work the deep neck flexors. To encourage lengthening while extending the back.

A subtle exercise that has dramatic results. It really does help to reverse the effects of being hunched over all day. You can feel the tension in your neck release as the shoulder blades slide down into your back.

## Starting Position

- Lie on your front with your forehead resting on the floor, feet hip-width apart and parallel.
- Create a diamond shape with your arms by placing your fingertips together just above your forehead.
- Your elbows are open, your shoulder blades relaxed.

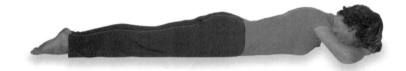

## Action

1 Breathe in, wide and full, and lengthen through the spine.

2 Breathe out, zip up and hollow – stay zipped and hollowed throughout the exercise – and glide the shoulder blades down toward the back of your waist.

3 Gently tuck your chin under as if holding a ripe peach, and raise your upper body one or two inches off the floor. Stay looking down at the floor. The back of your neck is long. Imagine a cord pulling you from the top of your head.

4 Really make the connection down into the small of your back – you have to push a little on the elbows, but think of them connecting with your waist as well.

5 Breathe in and hold the position. Keep the lower stomach lifted, with the ribs staying on the floor.

6 Breathe out and slowly lower back down. Keep lengthening through the spine.

7 Repeat six times.

## Watchpoints

- Keep the lower abdominals drawing back to the spine.
- Make sure you keep looking down at the floor – if you lift your head back you will shorten the back of the neck.

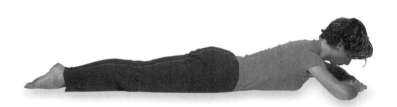

# The Dart: Stage Two

## Aim

To strengthen the back extensor muscles with trunk stability. To create awareness of the shoulder blades and to strengthen the muscles that stabilize them. To work the deep neck flexors.

This proceeds from what you learned in Stage One on page 77.

## Equipment

A small flat cushion (optional).

## Starting Position

- Lie on your front.
- You may place a flat cushion under your forehead to allow you to breathe.
- Your arms are down at your sides, your palms facing your body.
- Your neck is long.
- Your legs are together, parallel, with your toes softly pointed.

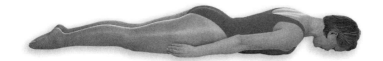

## Action

1 Breathe in, wide and full, to prepare, and lengthen through the spine, tucking your chin gently in as if to hold a ripe peach.

2 Breathe out, zip up and hollow – stay zipped and hollowed throughout the exercise – and glide your shoulder blades down into your back, lengthening your fingers away from you, down toward your feet, and turning the palms to face your body. The top of your head stays lengthening away from you. Tip your head back.

3 Gently squeeze your inner thighs together, but keep your feet on the floor and slowly raise the upper body.

4 Breathe in and feel the length of the body from the tips of your toes to the top of your head.

5 Breathe out, and lengthen and lower the upper body back down, releasing the lower body muscles.

6 Repeat eight times, then either roll on to your side or come back into the Rest Position (page 118).

## Watchpoints

• Keep hollowing the lower abdominals.

• Do not strain the neck. It should feel released as your shoulders engage down into your back. Think of a swan's neck extending out from between its wings.

• Remember to keep your feet on the floor.

• Stop if you feel at all uncomfortable in the low back.

• This exercise can also be done with the feet hip-width apart and the thigh and butt muscles relaxed.

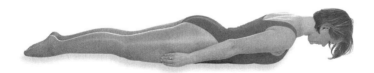

# Ankle Circles

## Aim

To free the ankle joint, increasing its mobility. To work the muscles, ligaments and tendons surrounding the ankle joint. To work the calf muscles.

For many of us, the muscles on the outer side of the ankle tend to be weak, which is why we are prone to sprained ankles when we "roll over" on the outside of the foot. This exercise is great for strengthening them.

## Equipment

A firm flat cushion (optional).

## Starting Position

- Lie in the Relaxation Position with your head on the cushion if it makes you more comfortable.
- Zip up and hollow and bend one knee up. Put your hands just behind the knee, with your thumbs coming around in front of it in order to be able to feel if your leg is moving.

## Action

1 Start to circle the foot very, very slowly and, taking it as far as you can, try to go to the maximum rotation. The leg should stay completely still, the movement coming totally from the ankle joint. Do not just wiggle your toes around.
2 Do five circles each way.

## Watchpoints

- What was happening to the rest of your body? Remember, shoulder blades down, breastbone soft, elbows open, lateral breathing, neutral pelvis.
- You do not need to zip up and hollow throughout this exercise, so use this as a break from stabilizing.

# Foot Exercises

## Aim

To reconnect the brain with the feet. To restore the arches of the feet. To mobilize the toes and their joints. To wake the feet up, increasing awareness to aid balance and proprioception. To work the muscles of the feet and the lower legs.

You may be wondering why we are including foot exercises in a book about backs, but the feet are very important to the health of the back. They are the foundation on which you stand; you would not consider building a house with unsound foundations! When standing, you need to think of a triangle or tripod on the sole of each foot. Mentally draw a triangle from the base of each big toe, to the base of the small toe to the center of the heel. You need to ground yourself on those two triangles with your weight evenly centered on them.

## Isolating the Toes

### Aim

To isolate the toes and learn control of the muscles of the foot.

### Equipment

A straight-backed chair (optional).

### Starting Position

- Stand or sit correctly (see page 66) in a chair with the feet flat on the floor.

### Action

1 Lift just the big toes off the floor; leave the others down!
2 Replace the big toes and reverse the action, lifting all the toes except for the big toe.

Can you do it? Keep practicing. You may cheat and use your fingers to move or hold the toes, but keep trying to do it properly. It's a great game at parties!

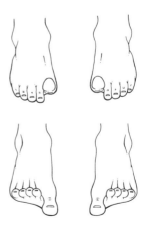

---

## The Mexican Wave

### Aim
To work the toes individually, re-awakening them.

### Starting Position and Equipment
Same as Isolating the Toes.

### Action
It's quite simple, really. One by one lift the toes, starting with the big toe, and "Mexican Wave" down to the little toe, then reverse the wave.

### Watchpoints for Isolating the Toes and the Mexican Wave
- Keep the bones at the base of your toes (the metatarsals) flat on the floor.
- Don't let the heels come off the floor.
- Don't let the feet roll.

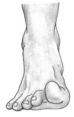 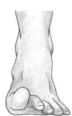

## Pointing and Flexing

### Aim
To learn how to point and flex the feet, while still maintaining good alignment in the rest of the legs. To work and stretch the flexors and extensors of the foot.

Many Pilates exercises require you to point or flex the feet.

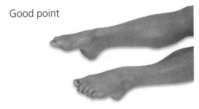

Good point

### Pointing
When pointing the foot or toes, point them softly. A very common mistake is to over-point so that the foot becomes "sickled" (shaped like a sickle). Instead, we want you to keep the front of the foot long and make sure the toes do not curl under.

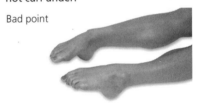

Bad point

### Flexing
When flexing the foot, push your heel away from your face. The toes will come up toward your face but, again, they do not curl over. Keep them long, the heel lengthening away.

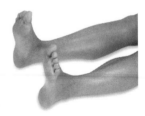

Good flex

# Working the Arches

## Aim

To strengthen the arches of the foot, helping to prevent flat feet.

Flat feet can change your whole postural stance, shortening the Achilles tendon and causing both upper- and lower-back imbalance. If the arches are weak, they will also contribute to the habit of rolling in the inside of the foot, upsetting the foundation on which good posture is built. The arches are the shock absorbers of the feet – they literally put the spring in our step.

## Equipment

A straight-backed chair (optional).

## Starting Position

- Sit on the floor with your knees bent, feet flat on the floor and parallel.
- Alternatively, you can simply stand correctly (see page 66) or sit on a chair with your feet on the floor, whichever is most comfortable.

## Action

1 Keeping the toes long and not letting them scrunch up, lift the inner borders of your feet, increasing the arches, drawing the bones at the base of the toes back toward the heel.
2 Hold for fifteen seconds then release.

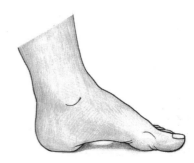

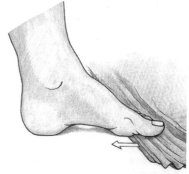

## Watchpoints

- Do not allow the feet to roll in or out.
- It's very tempting just to screw the toes up. That's not the idea, so make those arches work!
- If your foot cramps, rest and try again later.

# Deep Gluteal Stretch against the Wall

## Aim

To stretch the deep gluteals and the piriformis muscle.

This stretch can be very effective for those cases of sciatica that involve a tight piriformis muscle. Bear in mind, though, that there are many causes of sciatica.

The golden rule for Pilates is that you should never feel any pain at all. However, with some of the stretches like this one, it is quite normal to feel the stretch. This feeling shouldn't be painful – it should be deliciously unpleasant!

For the stretch to be effective, your tailbone must stay on the floor. It is an advanced stretch and, if you have limited flexibility in your hips, you will find even the starting position challenging. The Pelvic Stability Exercises on page 73 are a good preparation for it.

## Equipment

A firm flat cushion.

The deep butt muscles

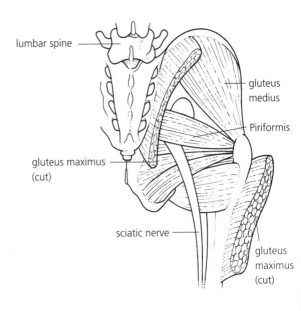

lumbar spine

gluteus medius

Piriformis

gluteus maximus (cut)

sciatic nerve

gluteus maximus (cut)

### Starting Position

- Get into the position shown in the photograph – it is easiest to approach the wall sideways and shuffle up as close as you can, then slowly swing the legs up the wall. You must still be comfortable.
- Rest your head on the cushion.
- Check that you are square on to the wall.
- For this exercise your butt should be six to eight inches from the wall.
- One leg is pointing straight up the wall.
- Rest the foot of the other leg just above the knee of the straight leg, turning the leg out from the hip joint so that the hip may open.
- Have your hands resting on your abdomen.

### Action

1 Slowly, slowly bend the straight leg, keeping it aligned. You will feel the stretch in the butt of the bent leg. The stretch will increase as you bend the leg more.
2 Keep your pelvis and spine in a neutral position. The tailbone will want to lift off the floor but you will lose the stretch if you allow it to.
3 Stay in this position for up to one minute, or until you feel the muscle release.
4 Repeat twice on each leg.

### Watchpoints

- Be aware of any discomfort in your back. Please do not continue if you feel pain in the lumbar area. You should feel the stretch in the butt of the bent knee.
- Keep checking that your tailbone has not lifted and that you have not twisted your pelvis. You must stay square to the wall.

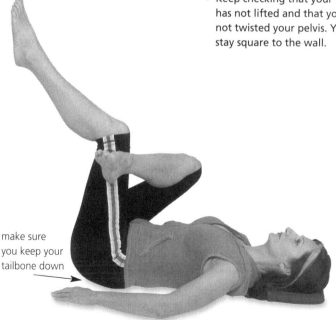

make sure you keep your tailbone down →

# The Monkey

## Aim

To learn how to protect the back by using the big joints, like the hip and knee. This is a vital exercise to help prevent backache and also strengthens the leg muscles. Once you have mastered this position, can do it with ease and have built endurance, you can perform many everyday actions that involve lifting or bending or standing without putting your back under stress.

## Starting Position

- Stand with your feet slightly turned out and hip-width apart.
- Your weight is evenly distributed between both feet and the spine is long.

## Action

1 Breathe in, wide and full, to prepare and lengthen the back.
2 Breathe out, zip up and hollow – stay zipped and hollowed throughout the exercise – and hinge your torso forward from the hip joint. Move the torso as one piece, including the head.
3 Breathe in while in this position.
4 Breathe out and bend your knees slightly over your feet and continue that hinging action of the torso.
5 Remain in this position for several breaths. Allow the back to widen and lengthen, and let the arms hang freely.
6 Keep the muscular tension in your legs minimal and keep lengthening your torso away from the legs.
7 After several breaths return slowly to standing, keeping your knees soft and the back lengthened.

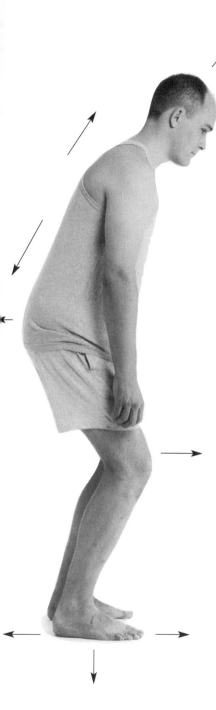

### Watchpoints

- It is as if you are zigzagging your legs under you. Keep the back in one piece and hinge from the hip joint.
- Don't be embarrassed to stick your butt out.
- Look at the arrows on the photograph and remember them when you are in the Monkey position.
- Keep your legs soft, and gradually increase the length of time you spend in this position. Initially it is very strenuous, but we promise that it gets easier!
- Remember this exercise especially when you are going to sit in a chair. This will make the transition from standing to sitting much smoother and avoid jarring the back.

# The Cat

## Aim

To mobilize the spine and learn correct alignment.

A wonderful exercise to help you move the spine bone by bone.

## Starting Position

- Kneel on all fours, your hands placed directly beneath your shoulders, the fingers facing forward. Your knees should be in line with your hips, the lower half of your legs straight. Look straight down at the floor so that the back of your neck is long.
- Find the natural, neutral curve in your spine and think of that small pool of water in the small of your back.
- Keep lengthening the top of your head away from your tailbone.
- Your shoulder blades should be down into your back.
- Do not be tempted to lock your elbows.
- Keep your weight on the whole of the hand, not just the heels.

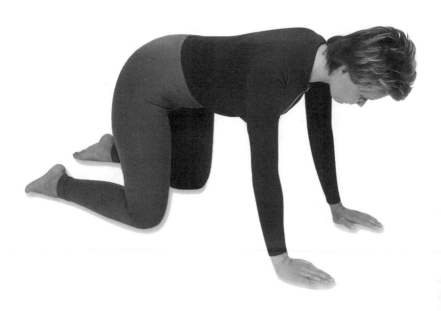

## Action

1 Breathe in, wide and full, to prepare, and lengthen through the spine.
2 Breathe out, zip up and hollow and stay zipped and hollowed throughout the exercise.
3 Start with the base of the spine and curl your tailbone under – a bit like you did for Spine Curls on page 91. Work your way up the spine, rounding it as you go, but keeping it open and wide. Your chin will end up on your chest, neck and head released. Imagine a hook pulling you from between the shoulder blades up to the ceiling.

4 Breathe in wide, checking that your elbows haven't locked.
5 Breathe out, and slowly uncurl the spine, starting again from the base, sticking your tailbone out, mobilizing vertebra by vertebra, sliding the shoulder blades down into your back, until you have returned to the Starting Position (i.e., neutral). Do not over-dip the low back or lift the head back. Feel the length of the spine.
6 Repeat five times.

## Watchpoints

- Keep the weight even on both hands.
- If your wrists tire, stop for a short break, then start again. Eventually they will strengthen.
- Focus on moving the spine bone by bone.
- Do not lock your elbows.

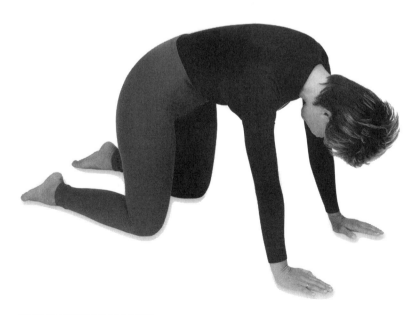

# Side-lying Quadriceps and Hip Flexor Stretch

## Aim

To stretch out the quadriceps, which run along the front of the thigh, and the hip flexors. To lengthen and iron out the front of the body, especially around the front of the hips, which can get very tight if you sit all day. To maintain good alignment of the torso by using the waist muscles and the shoulder stabilizers.

**Warning: Please seek advice if you have a knee injury. You may need to use a scarf to hook over the foot so that there is less pressure on the knee, or you may need to omit this exercise altogether.**

**There is a danger with this exercise that you may arch the back and stress the lumbar spine, so please take extra care in maintaining the neutral position of the pelvis. If in doubt, we would prefer you to play it safe and tuck the pelvis slightly under, that is, tilt it north.**

## Equipment

A scarf.
A firm flat cushion (optional).

## Starting Position

- Lie on your side with your head resting on your extended arm (you may like a flat cushion between the head and the arm to keep the neck in line).
- Have the knees bent at a right angle to your body.
- Your back should be in a straight line, but with its natural curve. Stack all your bones on top of each other – foot over foot, knee over knee, hip over hip and shoulder over shoulder.

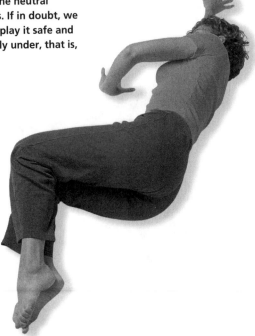

## Action

1 Breathe in, wide and full, to prepare and lengthen through the spine.
2 Breathe out, zip up and hollow – stay zipped and hollowed throughout the exercise – and bend the top knee toward you, taking hold of the front of the foot if you can reach it – you may need to use a scarf.
3 Breathe in and check your pelvic position. It should be neutral. (See **Warning** above.)
4 Breathe out and gently take the leg behind you to stretch the front of the thigh. Do not arch the back, keep the tailbone lengthening away from the top of your head. Think of the knee as lengthening away from the top of the head.
5 Hold the stretch for about twenty seconds, or until you feel the muscle release. Keep working the waist, which stays slightly lifted from the floor, keeping the length in the trunk.
6 After twenty seconds, slowly release by bringing the leg back in front of you.
7 Repeat three times on each side.

## Watchpoints

• Do not allow to knee to drop or lift; keep it in a line with the hip.
• Keep the waist long.
• Keep the shoulder blades down into the back and maintain the gap between the arms and the shoulders.
• Do not collapse forward. Keep the upper body open.
• If you cannot reach the foot in the stretch, or the stretch is too great and the knee feels stressed, try using the scarf wrapped over the front of the foot.

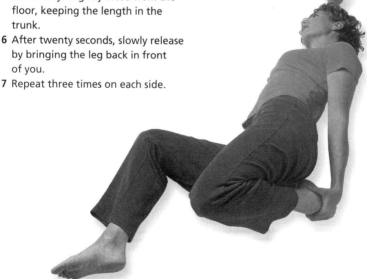

# Arm Openings

### Aim

To open the upper body and stretch the pectoral muscles, while stabilizing the shoulder blades. To achieve a sense of "openness" while stabilizing and centering. To rotate the spine gently and safely.

This has to be the most relaxing feel-good exercise in the Pilates program. Stay completely aware of your arm and hand as they displace the air, moving through space.

**Warning: Since this exercise involves rotation of the spine, seek advice if you have a disc-related injury.**

### Equipment

A firm flat cushion.
A tennis ball (optional).

### Starting Position

- Lie on your side with your head on a cushion, knees curled up at a right angle to your body. Your back should be in a straight line, but with its natural curve.
- Place a tennis ball between the knees (the idea is that the tennis ball keeps your knees and pelvis in good alignment).
- Line all your bones on top of each other – feet, ankles, knees, hips and shoulders.
- Your arms are extended in front of you, palms together at shoulder height.

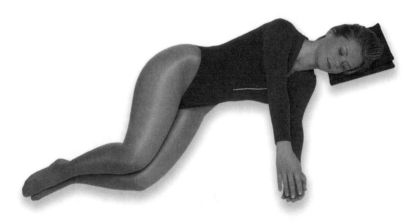

## Action

1 Breathe in to prepare and lengthen through the spine.
2 Breathe out, zip up and hollow and stay zipped and hollowed throughout the exercise.
3 Breathe in as you slowly extend and lift the upper arm, keeping the elbow soft and the shoulder blade down into the back. Keep your eyes on your hand so that your head follows the arm movement. You are aiming to touch the floor behind you, but do not force it.
4 Try to keep your knees together, your pelvis still.
5 Breathe out as you bring the arm back in an arc to rest on the other hand again.
6 Repeat five times, then curl up on the other side and start again.

## Watchpoints

• Keep hollowing throughout.
• Keep your waist long. Do not allow it to sink into the floor.
• Don't forget to allow your head to roll naturally with the movement, but do make sure that it is supported by the cushion.
• Keep the gap between your ears and your shoulders by engaging the muscles below the shoulder blades.

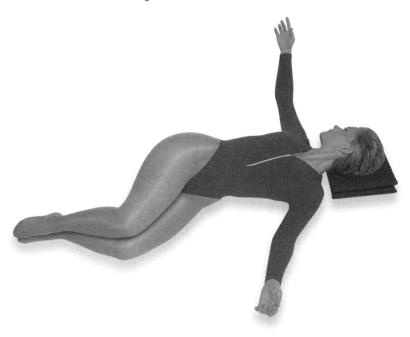

# The Cushion Squeeze

## Aim

To isolate and work the pelvic floor in conjunction with the deep abdominals, engaging the deep stabilizers. To strengthen the inner thighs (adductors). To learn the correct position of the pelvis. To open the lower back.

This is a great exercise if you suffer from the kind of sciatica that is caused by an overactive piriformis muscle.

## Equipment

A firm flat cushion (optional).
A plump cushion.

## Starting Position

- Lie in the Relaxation Position, with your head on the flat cushion if it makes you more comfortable, but have your feet together flat on the floor.
- Place a plump cushion between your knees. If you have sciatica, place it between your thighs near your knees.
- Check that your pelvis is in neutral.

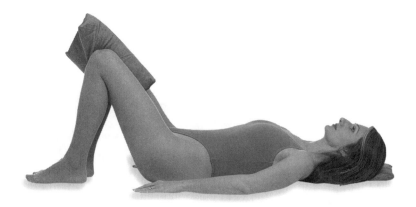

## Action

1 Breathe in, wide and full, to prepare.
2 Breathe out and zip up and hollow. Squeeze the cushion between your knees. Keep the pelvis in neutral, the tailbone down on the floor, lengthening away. Try not to grip around the hips.
3 Continue to breathe normally, squeezing and working the pelvic floor and deep abdominals, for a count of up to ten. Then release.
4 Repeat five times.

## Watchpoints

• Do not hold your breath – keep breathing.
• Keep your neck released and your jaw soft. You do not need to use your neck to work the pelvic floor.
• The most common mistake made doing this exercise is lifting the tailbone and tucking the pelvis. Think of keeping the length in the front of the pelvis; do not curl or shorten it. Another good way to check if you are tilting is to place your hand under your waist. Do the exercise wrong initially, tucking the pelvis, and feel the pressure on your hand as you push into the spine. Now try to do the exercise with no pressure on the hand – you have stayed in neutral.

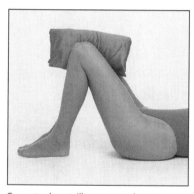

Correct when tailbone stays down

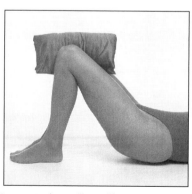

Incorrect when tailbone lifts

# Stage Three

# Outer Circle: Challenge it!

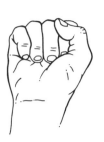

# The Pelvic Bridge

## Aim

To learn pelvic stability and to strengthen the butt.

This isn't as easy as it looks and requires good abdominals and back muscles. If you find yourself wobbling, you may not be ready yet, so practice the exercises in the Middle Circle for a while longer.

## Equipment

A firm flat cushion (optional).

## Starting Position

- Lie in the Relaxation Position, with your head on the cushion if it makes you more comfortable, your feet about eight inches from your butt.
- Unlike normal Spine Curls, place your feet together (line up the bunions!).
- Leave your arms down by your sides, palms down.

## Action

1 Breathe in, wide and full, to prepare.
2 Breathe out, zip up and hollow and slowly lift your lower body from the floor, keeping your pelvis in neutral.
3 Breathe normally as you check that your spine is now in a neutral position and bring your hands to rest on your pelvis.

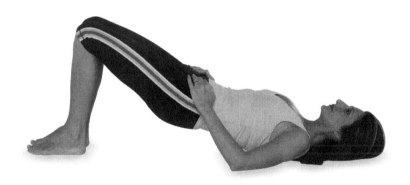

4 On your next out breath, still zipping and hollowing, straighten one leg, keeping the knees together so that the leg extends in a straight line. Keep your pelvis completely still; do not allow it to dip. Think of keeping both sides of your waist long.

5 Breathe in and return the foot to the floor.

6 Work up to repeating the exercise twenty times with each leg before lowering your body back down on to the floor.

**Watchpoints**

• There is a tendency sometimes, when there is a muscle imbalance in the torso, for one side to dominate. As you lift and lower the spine think of a jet taking off and landing right down the central strip of the runway. No high cross wind, please!

• Keep checking constantly that, as you extend your leg, your pelvis stays in neutral north and south, east and west.

• Use your hands to check for movement in the pelvis. They will also automatically help to keep you a little more stable.

*Moving On*
To make this exercise harder, take your hands away from your pelvis and fold them easily across your chest. This reduces your base of support, which means that you have to work harder to stabilize.

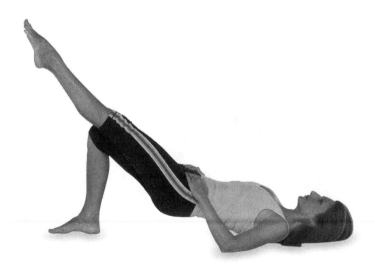

# Roll Downs

## Roll Downs against the Wall

We have given you two versions here. You should master the first one using the wall and be comfortable with it before you attempt the free-standing version.

### Aim
To release tension in the spine, the shoulders and the upper body. To mobilize the spine, creating flexibility and strength and achieving segmental control. To teach correct use of stabilizing abdominals when bending.

A core exercise in any Pilates program, this can be used as a warm-up or a wind-down. It combines stabilizing work with the wonderful wheeling motion of the spine.

As you roll back up, think of rebuilding the spinal column, stacking the vertebrae on top of each other to lengthen out the spine.

**Warning: Seek advice if you have a back problem (see Action, point 3, below), especially if it is disc-related.**

### Starting Position
- Stand about eighteen inches from a wall (the distance really depends on your height, but you should feel comfortable).
- Your knees are bent so that from the side you look as if you are sitting on a bar stool.
- Have your feet hip-width apart and parallel, your weight evenly balanced on both feet. Check that you are not rolling your feet in or out.
- Find your neutral pelvis position, but keep the tailbone lengthening down.

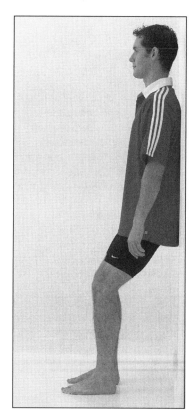

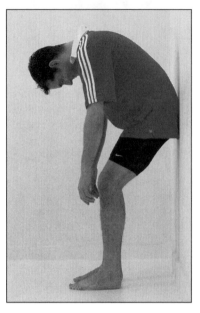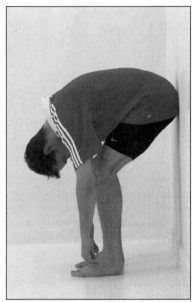

## Action

1 Breathe in to prepare and lengthen up through the spine; release the head and neck.

2 Breathe out, zip up and hollow and stay zipped and hollowed throughout the exercise. Drop your chin to your chest and allow the weight of your head to make you slowly roll forward, head released, arms hanging, center strong, knees soft.

3 If you have a back problem, you may like to begin by sliding your hands down your thighs.

4 Breathe in as you hang, really letting your head and arms hang down.

5 Breathe out, firmly zipped up and hollowed, as you drop your tailbone down, directing your pubic bone forward. Rotate your pelvis backward as you slowly come up the wall, rolling through the spine bone by bone.

6 Repeat six times.

## Watchpoints

• You may like to take an extra breath during the exercise. This is fine, but please try to breathe out as you move the spine.

• Make sure that you go down centrally and do not sway over to one side. When you are down, check where your hands are in relation to your feet.

• Do not roll the feet in or out. Keep the weight evenly balanced and try not to lean forward on to the front of your feet or back on to your heels.

# Free-standing Roll Downs

## Starting Position

- Stand with your feet hip-width apart and parallel, your weight evenly balanced on both feet. Check that you are not rolling your feet in or out.
- Soften your knees.
- Find your neutral pelvis position, but keep the tailbone lengthening down.

## Action

**1** Breathe in to prepare and lengthen up through the spine; release the head and neck.

**2** Breathe out, zip up and hollow – stay zipped and hollowed throughout the exercise – and drop your chin on to your chest and allow the weight of your head to make you slowly roll forward, head released, arms hanging, center strong, knees soft.

**3** Breathe in as you hang, really letting your head and arms hang down.

**4** Breathe out, firmly zipped, as you drop your tailbone down, directing your pubic bone forward. Rotate your pelvis backward as you slowly come up to standing tall, rolling through the spine bone by bone.

**5** Repeat six times.

### Watchpoints

- You may like to take an extra breath during the exercise. This is fine, but please try to breathe out as you move the spine.
- Make sure that you go down centrally and that you do not sway over to one side. When you are down, check where your hands are in relation to your feet.
- Do not roll the feet in or out. Keep the weight evenly balanced and try not to lean forward on to the front of your feet or back on your heels.

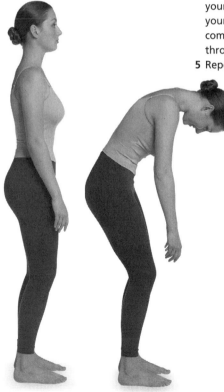

# Hip Rolls with Shoulder Blade Setting

### Aim

To stretch and work the waist (quadratus lumborum) and to strengthen the oblique abdominals. To achieve a safe rotation of the spine with segmental control. To promote awareness of the shoulder blades using the stabilizing muscles. To learn coordination skills.

We are looking here for rotation with stability. The ability to rotate the spine is the first movement we tend to lose as we grow older. There is a lot to think about with this exercise, which is great since we are trying to train the mind as well as the body! Focus on:

- Using the lower abdominals throughout.
- Peeling each part of your back off the floor in turn – first your butt leaves the floor, then the hips, the waist and finally the back of the ribs. Then as you return to the center, place each part back on the floor in reverse order – the ribs, the waist, the hips, the butt.

- As you turn the palm down, think of the shoulder blade setting itself down into your back.

**Warning: Please seek advice if you have a disc-related injury. If you have had a whiplash injury, keep your head in the center.**

### Equipment

A tennis ball. This helps you keep good leg and pelvic alignment.

### Starting Position

- Lie on your back, arms out to the side, palms up.
- Your knees should be up toward your chest, but in line with your hips.
- Place the tennis ball between your knees.
- Your thighs will be at right angles to your body.
- Your feet are softly pointed.

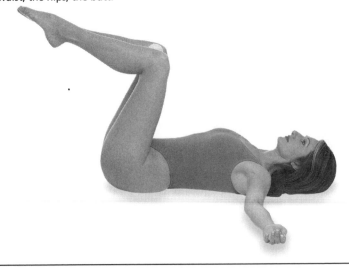

## Action

1 Breathe in, wide and full, to prepare. As you breathe out, zip up and hollow – stay zipped and hollowed throughout the exercise – and slowly lower your legs toward the floor on your right side, turning your head to the left. Keep the left shoulder and palm down on the ground. Keep the knees in line.

2 Breathe in and breathe out and use your strong center to bring your legs back to the middle. At the same time return the head to the middle and turn the palm up.

3 Breathe in and then out, and repeat the twisting movement to the opposite side.

4 Repeat ten times to each side.

## Watchpoints

- Keep the opposite shoulder firmly down on the floor.
- Keep the knees in line. Don't go too far unless you can control it.
- Use the abdominals at all times – feel as though you are moving the legs using the abdominals.
- It is a sideways lateral movement – don't deviate.
- Do not force the neck the opposite way. Allow it to roll comfortably and keep it long.

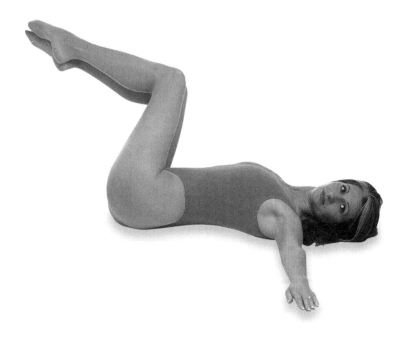

# Butt Scrunches

## Aim

To strengthen the gluteals.

The good news is this is a great butt-toning exercise!

## Starting Position

- Lie on your front in a straight line.
- Rest your forehead on your folded hands.
- Your legs are parallel.
- Your upper body should remain relaxed throughout the exercise.

## Action

1 Breathe in, wide and full, to prepare, and lengthen through the spine.
2 Breathe out, zip up and hollow – stay zipped and hollowed throughout the exercise – and bend one knee, bringing the calf toward the back of your thigh at an angle of about 90°.
3 Breathe in, wide and full, again.
4 Breathe out, and slowly lift the thigh just a little from the floor – it will only move about 10° maximum.
5 Keep your pelvis still, with the weight evenly distributed between both hip joints. Do not allow your low back to dip; use your zip up and hollow to support your lumbar spine. Try not to use the hamstrings at the back of your leg to lift the leg – try to use your butt muscles instead.
6 Breathe normally and hold the leg there for a count of three before slowly lowering.
7 Repeat three times with each leg.

**Watchpoints**
- Keep the hip joints on the floor.
- Keep zipping and hollowing and lengthening through the spine.
- Keep your upper body relaxed.
- Try not to use the non-working leg.

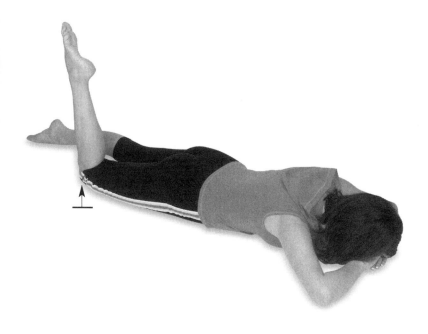

# Full Table Top

## Aim

To learn how to keep your center stabilized while moving the limbs, maintaining neutral and keeping the length in the trunk. To learn balance and control. To learn pelvic stability and to work the deep gluteals.

The key to this exercise is keeping your girdle of strength working, supporting the spine and keeping both sides of the waist long, the pelvis neutral and level. No tension should creep into the upper body.

You must be able to do the simpler versions of this exercise on page 134 before you move on to this more challenging version.

A complementary exercise would be Standing on One Leg and the Oyster on pages 132 and 112.

## Stage One

### Starting Position

- Kneel on all fours, your hands directly beneath your shoulders, your knees beneath your hips.
- Check that your pelvis is neutral, the natural curve of your back maintained.

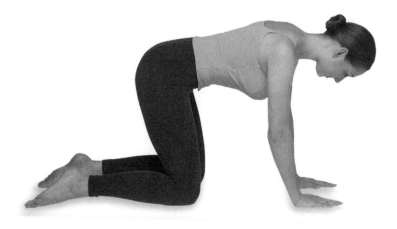

## Action

1 Breathe in, wide and full, to prepare, as you lengthen the spine from the top of your head to your tailbone.

2 Breathe out, zip up and hollow – stay zipped and hollowed throughout the exercise – and slide the right leg away from you, straightening it along the floor.

3 Breathe in and then out as you slowly lift the leg to hip height – no higher! The pelvis must stay absolutely level; do not allow the low back to dip.

4 As you lift the leg on the out breath, simultaneously lift and lengthen the opposite arm to shoulder height. Do not overreach. Keep the shoulder blade down and the neck long. The pelvis stays square to the floor.

5 Keep looking at the floor with the top of the head lengthening away from the tailbone.

6 Breathe in and lower the arm and leg.

7 Repeat five times, alternating arms and legs.

## Watchpoints

• Keep the lower abdominals engaged throughout.

• Do not allow the pelvis to tilt to one side.

• Keep looking straight down at the floor – if you raise your head, you will shorten the back of your neck.

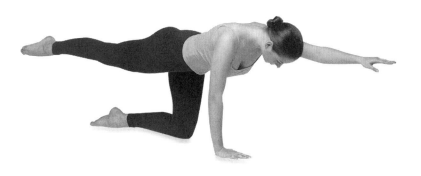

# The Torpedo

## Aim

This is one of the hardest exercises in this book. You need very strong core stabilizing muscles and very good body awareness. It strengthens the muscles of your waist.

## Equipment

A small flat cushion (optional).

## Starting Position

- Lie in a straight line on your side – double-check, or get someone else to, that you are straight: shoulder over shoulder, hip over hip, pelvis in neutral.
- The underneath arm is under your head and in line with your body. You might find it more comfortable if you have a cushion between your head and your arm.
- Your legs are stretched out and in a line with your body.
- Your upper arm stays in front of the body with the hand opposite the chest on the floor, fingers parallel to the torso.
- Keep your shoulder blades down and the upper body relaxed, but not collapsed.

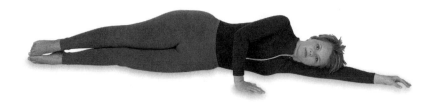

## Action

1 Breathe in to prepare, and lengthen the back.

2 Breathe out, zip up and hollow and stay zipped and hollowed throughout the exercise.

3 Breathing in, lift both legs together off the mat.

4 Breathing out, keep the underneath leg up and raise the upper leg further, keeping it parallel to the lower leg.

5 Keep your pelvis in neutral and keep your center strong.

6 Breathing in, bring the legs together.

7 Normally the top leg is lowered to the stationary leg underneath, but the latter has often dropped, so this exercise is usually taught moving both to work the abductors fully.

8 Breathing out, lower the legs gently to the floor, maintaining a long waistline.

## Watchpoints

• Good core stability is the key to balance. Try not to use the supporting arm.

• Check your alignment constantly – do not let your back arch.

• Keep your legs parallel.

• The supporting arm and shoulder should have the elbow open, the shoulder blade down.

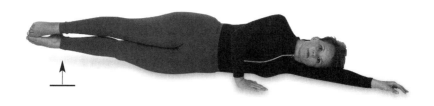

# One-legged Calf Raises

## Aim

To learn to move with a balanced pelvis, while on one leg. To strengthen the calf muscles and activate the calf pump.

## Starting Position

- Stand alongside to a wall, lengthening through the spine. You may hold on to the wall for support.
- Zip up and hollow and bend the knee of the leg closest to the wall. The knee faces straight forward and the calf rests beside the weight-bearing knee.
- The pelvis stays still, and the hip bones are level.

## Action

1 Breathe in, wide and full, to prepare, and lengthen up through the spine.
2 Breathe out, zip up and hollow – stay zipped and hollowed throughout the exercise – and rise up on your toes.
3 Breathe in.
4 Breathe out, and slowly return heel to the floor.
5 Breathe in, wide and full.
6 Breathe out, and slowly bend the knee directly over the center of the foot, keeping the heel down. Do not bend too far; maintain control.
7 Breathe in and straighten.
8 Repeat up to ten times with each leg.

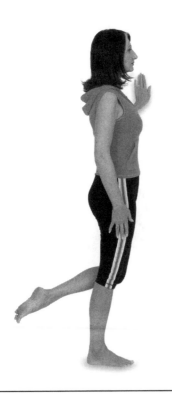 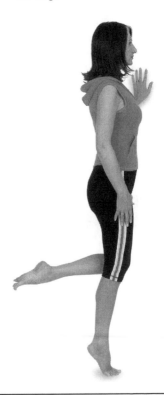

## Watchpoints

- Work slowly through the foot, and do not let the ankle twist in or out.
- The movement should not alter your overall alignment. Pay particular attention to balancing the head, ribcage and pelvis over each other.
- Do not allow your butt to stick out, and try not to pitch forward.

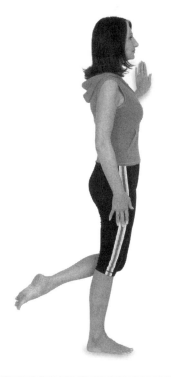
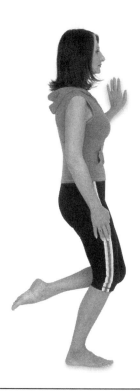

# Abductor Lifts

## Aim

To strengthen the outer thigh (abductors) and the butt (gluteals). To tone the upper leg and control cellulite.

This exercise and Adductor Lifts (page 176) will challenge your pelvic and lumbar stability, so you must be stable before you attempt them. Good preparation exercises are the Pelvic Stability Exercises (pages 73), Standing on One Leg (pages 132) and Table Top: Stages One and Two (pages 134).

You may want to perform this exercise and the two following exercises on one side before turning to the other side.

## Equipment

First practice these exercises without weights until you are totally familiar with them and they cause you no discomfort. You may then strap leg weights of up to three pounds on each ankle. Start with the lightest weight.

A cushion (optional).

A small piece of foam (optional).

## Starting Position

- Lie on your left side in a straight line. This is crucial, so, if you'd like, you can lie up against a wall to check your alignment. Don't lean against the wall.
- Remember, neutral, please.
- Your left arm is stretched out with your head resting on the arm. You may place a cushion between your ear and your arm so that the head is in line with the spine.
- Bend both legs in front of you to an angle of just under 90°.
- Put your right hand in front of your body to help support you.
- Throughout the exercise, keep lifting the waist off the floor and maintaining the length in the trunk.

## Action

1 Zip up and hollow and stay zipped and hollowed throughout the exercise.

2 Straighten your top leg so that it is in a line with your hip, and raise it to about five inches off the floor. Be careful not to take it behind you.

3 Rotate the leg inward slightly from the hip, the pelvis staying still, and flex the foot toward your face. You should be able to see your toes.

4 Breathe out as you slowly lift the leg higher to about six inches, then breathe in and lower.

5 Raise and lower the leg ten times without returning it to the floor. Breathe out as you raise and in as you lower.

6 Bend the leg and rest it on the lower leg.

7 Repeat on each side.

## Watchpoints

• Keep zipping and hollowing so you protect the low back and prevent it from arching. Keep the waist from dropping down to the floor.

• Lengthen the heel as far away as possible from the hip – keep a long, long leg.

• Keep the rotation inward from the hip, being careful not to turn it in just from the ankle.

• Keep lifting the waist off the floor and lengthening in the body – long, long waist.

• Your pelvis should remain absolutely still. Do not allow it to roll forward or rock around.

• Don't forget to keep the upper body open, shoulder blades down into your back. Do not allow yourself to roll forward.

NOTE If you are lucky enough to lack any natural padding around your hip, you may find it uncomfortable to lie like this. If so, just put a small piece of foam underneath your hip.

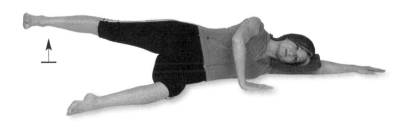

# Adductor Lifts

## Aim

To tone the inner thigh (adductor) muscles. To learn pelvic stability.

## Equipment

First practice these exercises without weights until you are totally familiar with them and they cause you no discomfort. You may then strap leg weights of up to three pounds on each ankle. Start with the lightest weight.

A large cushion.

## Starting Position

- Lie on your left side, as for the Abductor Lifts.
- Keeping your bottom leg straight, bend the knee of your upper leg and rest it on top of a large cushion. The idea is that your pelvis stays square and does not drop forward.
- Stretch the bottom leg away a little in front of you, turning it out from the hip joint.
- Point or flex the foot, either is fine.

## Action

1 Breathe in, wide and full, to prepare.
2 Keep the leg turned out from the hip, long and straight.
3 Breathe out and zip up and hollow – stay zipped and hollowed throughout the exercise – as you slowly raise the underneath leg. Keep lengthening it away.
4 Do not allow your waist to sink into the floor; keep working it.
5 Breathe in as you lower the leg.
6 Repeat up to twenty times on each side.

## Watchpoints

- Keep zipping and hollowing throughout.
- Don't let your waist sag; keep lengthening it.
- Check that you are moving the whole leg together and not just twisting from the knee.
- Don't let your foot sickle (curl) around to help you come up further; the action must be from the inside of the thigh.
- Check that your upper body stays open, shoulder blades down. Do not roll forward.

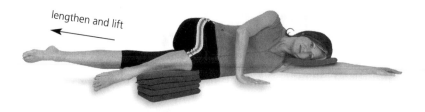

lengthen and lift

# Backstroke Swimming

## Aim
To learn correct shoulder movement, stabilizing the scapulae. To open the shoulder blades. To combat round shoulders. To work the adductors.

A wonderful exercise to counter those hunched positions that we all find ourselves in every day. Enjoy the sensation of opening out.

## Equipment
A firm flat cushion (optional).
A tennis ball or plump cushion.
Hand-weights of between one and two pounds each.

## Starting Position
- With this exercise, try to remember the movement pattern you learned in the Starfish on page 82.
- Lie on a narrow bench, if possible, in the Relaxation Position, with your head on the firm cushion if it makes you more comfortable, but this time bring your feet together flat on the floor, with your legs parallel to each other.
- Put a tennis ball or a cushion between the knees.
- Holding the hand weights, raise your arms to the ceiling, your palms away from your face, your elbows slightly bent.

- Throughout the exercise stay zipped up and hollowed and gently squeeze the cushion or tennis ball.
- Remember to stay in neutral.

## Action
1 Breathe in, wide and full, to prepare.
2 Breathe out and zip up and hollow as you take the right arm behind you to the floor, if that is possible; otherwise; as far as is comfortable, while the left hand moves down to the side of your hip and you squeeze the cushion between your knees.
3 Keep your ribcage calm, your shoulder blades down into your back, and maintain a gap between your ears and your shoulders.
4 Breathe in as you bring the arms back up to the Starting Position.
5 Breathe out as you repeat the movement to the other side.
6 Keep squeezing the tennis ball and hollowing the lower abdominals.
7 Repeat ten times on each side.

## Watchpoints
- Do not overreach with the arms; keep the elbows slightly bent.
- Do not force the arm back.

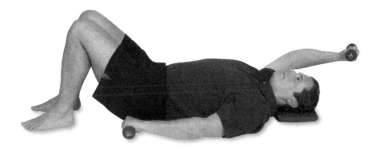

# Single Leg Stretch

## Aim

This is a classic Pilates exercise, which is best taught in simple stages. It challenges both the abdominals and your coordination. In fact, it combines *all* the Eight Principles.

## Stage One

### Equipment

A firm flat cushion (optional).

### Starting Position

- Lie in the Relaxation Position, with your head on the cushion if it makes you more comfortable.

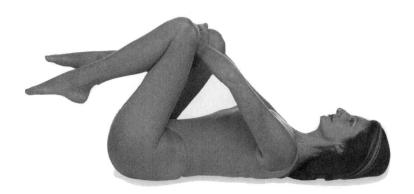

## Action

1 Breathe in, wide and full, to prepare.

2 Breathe out, zip up and hollow – stay zipped and hollowed throughout the exercise – and fold one knee at a time up toward your chest.

3 Breathe in, and with both hands hold your left leg under the thigh. Keep your elbows open and your breastbone soft. Your shoulder blades stay down into your back. Your neck is released.

4 Breathe out and slowly straighten the right leg up into the air. Keep your back anchored into the floor.

5 Breathe in and bend the knee back in.

6 Take hold of the other leg and repeat the exercise.

7 Repeat ten times with each leg.

8 Do not allow the leg to fall away from you. Your back must stay anchored to the floor.

9 When this becomes easy – and only when – you may try the more advanced version on the next page.

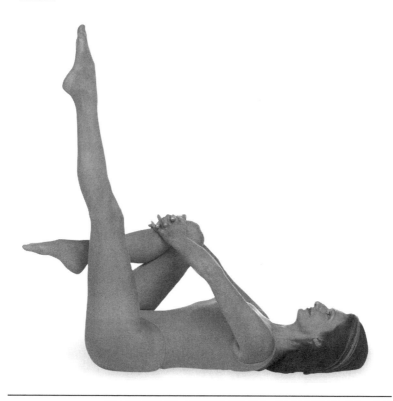

## Stage Two

This has to be the best abdominal exercise there is!

### Equipment and Starting Position
Same as Stage One.

### Action

1 Breathe in to prepare.
2 Breathe out, zip up and hollow and fold your knees up toward your chest one at a time. The toes are just touching but the heels aren't so the legs are open. Keep your feet softly pointed. Place your hands on the outside of your calves.
3 Breathe in, checking that your elbows are open to enable the chest to expand fully. Your shoulder blades are down into your back.
4 Breathe out, zip up and hollow – stay zipped and hollowed throughout the exercise – and soften your breastbone and curl the upper body off the floor.

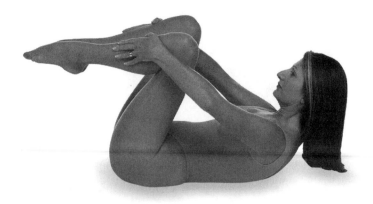

5 Breathe in and place the right hand on the outside of the right ankle, the left hand on the inside of the right knee.

6 Breathe out and slowly stretch your left leg away parallel so that it is at an angle of 45° to the floor. The toes are softly pointed.

7 Breathe in, wide and full, as you begin to bend the leg back on to your chest, bringing it back toward your shoulder.

8 Change hands, so that your left hand is on the outside of your left leg, your right hand on the inside of your left knee.

9 Breathe out and stretch the right leg away, keeping it parallel. Do not take it too close to the floor.

10 Breathe in as the leg returns.

11 Repeat ten stretches on each leg, making sure that you have a strong center throughout, that your shoulder blades stay down into your back and that your elbows are open.

## Watchpoints

- Keep zipping and hollowing throughout, and do not allow the back to arch. The pelvis stays neutral.
- Keep your neck released and the upper body open, your shoulder blades down.
- Make sure that you keep the length on both sides of your waist – do not allow one side to shorten.

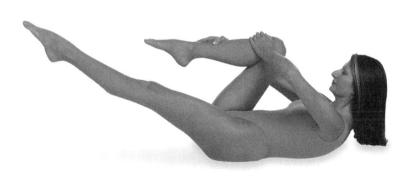

# The Hundred: Stages One to Four

## Aim

To learn lateral lower ribcage breathing to a set rhythm. To strengthen the pectoral muscles. To master stabilizing the shoulder blades. To strengthen the abdominals.

The Hundred is one of the classic Pilates exercises. It used to be the warm-up exercise for mat classes and it certainly does warm you up. We have broken the exercise down into manageable chunks. When you have mastered one stage, then – and only then – you may proceed to the next. This first stage tackles the breathing pattern, which stimulates the circulatory system, oxygenating the blood.

## Stage One

### Equipment for All Stages

A firm flat cushion (optional).

### Breathing Preparation

- Lie in the Relaxation Position, with your head on the cushion if it makes you more comfortable.
- Place your hands on your lower ribcage.
- Breathe in, wide and full, into your sides and back for a count of five.
- Breathe out and zip up and hollow for a count of five.
- Repeat ten times, trying to stay zipped and hollowed for both the in and out breaths.
- If you find the count of five too difficult, try a count of three.

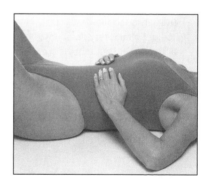

# Stage Two

## Starting Position

- Lie in the Relaxation Position, with your head on the cushion if it makes you more comfortable.
- Zip up and hollow and bend your knees up toward your chest one at a time. Your legs are parallel to each other.
- Your arms are extended alongside your body, palms down, wrists straight.
- Leave your head down on the floor.

## Action

1 Breathing in wide into your sides and back, pump your arms up and down, no more than six inches off the floor for a count of three. The shoulder blades stay down with the fingers lengthening away.
2 Breathe out and pump the arms for a count of three.
3 Repeat ten times.
4 When this breathing pattern is familiar to you and you are able to coordinate it with the pumping arm movement, try breathing in for five beats and out for five beats. Work up to twenty repetitions, hence the Hundred.

## Watchpoints

- Your breathing should be comfortable. Do not "over breathe." If you feel lightheaded, take a break.
- As you beat the arms, be aware of any unnecessary tension in your neck. Keep the neck released.
- Your shoulder blades should stay down into your back as your arms lengthen away.

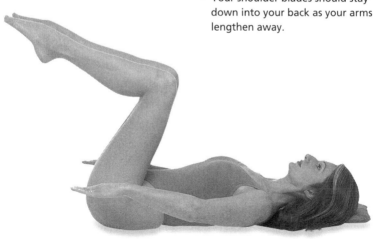

## Stage Three

### Aim

To add abdominal training to the breathing. To work the deep neck flexors while keeping the superficial neck muscles released.

**Warning: Please seek advice if you have neck, respiratory or heart problems.**

### Starting Position

- Lie in the Relaxation Position, with your head on the cushion if it makes you more comfortable.
- Zip up and hollow and bring your knees up toward your chest one at a time, keeping the legs parallel.
- Your toes are softly pointed, your arms down by your side.
- Slowly roll your head from side to side to release your neck.

### Action

1 Breathe in, wide and full, to prepare.
2 Breathe out, zip up and hollow – stay zipped and hollowed throughout the exercise – and curl the upper body off the floor, remembering everything you learned for Curl Ups (page 120). Your chin is gently tucked forward as if you are holding a ripe peach, jaw relaxed, soft breastbone, released neck.
3 Start the breathing and pumping action of the arms that you mastered in the last stage. Breathe in laterally for five beats and out for five beats.
4 Keep the shoulder blades down and a large gap between your ears and your shoulders. Keep reaching away with your fingers.
5 Repeat twenty times until you reach a hundred, then slowly, still zipped and hollowed, return the feet to the floor one at a time.

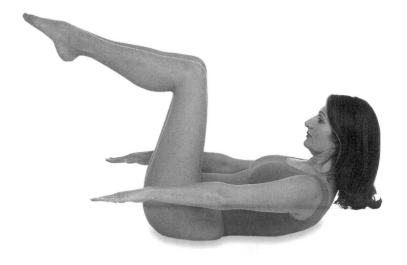

# Stage Four

## Watchpoints

- Return to the floor if you feel any strain at all in your neck.
- To prevent strain and to engage the deep stabilizers, have your chin gently tucked in but not squashed. Your line of sight should be between your knees. The back of your neck remains long, the front relaxed.
- You must keep breathing wide into your lower ribcage or you will become breathless. If you do feel breathless, stop at once!
- Keep a sense of width in your upper body. Do not close the shoulders in; keep the upper body open, the breastbone soft.

## Starting Position

Same as Stage Three.

## Action

1 When you are really strong follow Actions 1 and 2 in Stage Three but, this time, slowly straighten the legs into the air as far as is comfortable.
2 Do not allow your legs to fall away from you; your back must stay anchored and in neutral.
3 The toes are softly pointed.
4 Breathe in and out and pump the arms for a count of a hundred before bending the knees and lowering the legs one at a time to the floor.

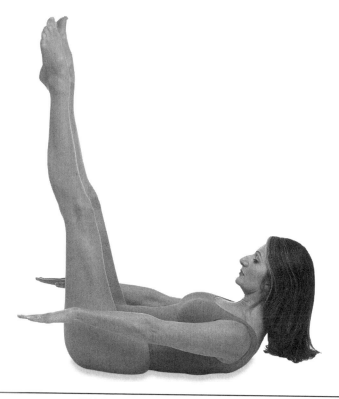

# Recommended Workouts

How often should you exercise? Which exercises should you do? If you have a back problem, then ideally you should do a minimum of twenty minutes exercise each and every day to help you re-balance the body and establish sound movement patterns. When you have more time you can attempt the longer workouts. Aim to do at least three hours' exercise per week.

Please remember that the Pilates Back-training Program is non-aerobic, so you will also need to include some aerobic sessions in your fitness plan.

We have provided here a selection of balanced workouts of varying lengths. Remember that it is far better to do a few exercises well than attempt to do too many and rush them. Simply do fewer repetitions if you have less time.

# Workouts from Stages One and Two: The Inner and Middle Circles

Please note that these are daily work-outs. When you are very familiar with the exercises they will take you about twenty minutes.

**Day 1**

| | | |
|---|---|---|
| 1 The Relaxation Position | p. 61 | |
| 2 Lateral Breathing | p. 67 | |
| 3 Pelvic Stability Exercises – choose any two | p. 73 | |
| 4 The Starfish | p. 82 | |
| 5 Hip Flexor Stretch | p. 94 | |
| 6 Spine Curls | p. 91 | |
| 7 Side Rolls | p. 95 | |
| 8 Neck Rolls and Chin Tucks | p. 84 | |
| 9 Curl Ups | p. 120 | |
| 10 Oblique Curl Ups | p. 121 | |
| 11 The Dart: Stage Two | p. 138 | |
| 12 The Star | p. 115 | |
| 13 The Cat | p. 148 | |
| 14 The Rest Position | p. 118 | |
| 15 The Oyster | p. 112 | |
| 16 Shoulder Drops | p. 86 | |
| 17 The Cushion Squeeze | p. 154 | |

**Day 2**

|  |  | |
|---|---|---|
| 1 Alignment in Standing with the Pelvic Elevator | p. 66 | |
| 2 Walking on the Spot plus Calf Stretch | p. 101 | |
| 3 Arm Circles against the Wall | p. 103 | |
| 4 Dumb Waiter on the Wall | p. 108 | |
| 5 Pelvic Stability Exercises – choose any two | p. 73 | |
| 6 Knee Circles with Breath | p. 97 | |
| 7 Hamstring Stretch | p. 122 | |
| 8 Neck Rolls and Chin Tucks | p. 84 | |
| 9 Curl Ups | p. 120 | |
| 10 The Diamond Press | p. 136 | |
| 11 The Big Squeeze | p. 114 | |
| 12 Knee Swings | p. 110 | |
| 13 Table Top: Stage One | p. 134 | |
| 14 The Rest Position | p. 118 | |
| 15 Adductor Openings | p. 124 | |
| 16 Side-lying Quadriceps and Hip Flexor Stretch | p. 150 | |
| 17 Arm Openings | p. 152 | |

## Day 3

|  |  | |
|---|---|---|
| 1 The Starfish 🖐 | p. 82 | |
| 2 Spine Curls ✌ | p. 91 | |
| 3 Hip Flexor Stretch ✌ | p. 94 | |
| 4 Windmill Arms ✌ | p. 99 | |
| 5 Neck Rolls and Chin Tucks 🖐 | p. 84 | |
| 6 Oblique Curl Ups ✌ | p. 121 | |
| 7 Ankle Circles ✌ | p. 140 | |
| 8 Adductor Openings ✌ | p. 124 | |
| 9 The Oyster ✌ | p. 112 | |
| 10 Deep Gluteal Stretch against the Wall ✌ | p. 144 | |
| 11 The Dart: Stage Two ✌ | p. 138 | |
| 12 The Cat ✌ | p. 148 | |
| 13 The Rest Position ✌ | p. 118 | |
| 14 Sitting or Standing Waist Twists ✌ | p. 130 or p.131 | |
| 15 Floating Arms 🖐 | p. 79 | |
| 16 Chicken Wings on the Wall ✌ | p. 126 | |
| 17 Walking on the Spot plus Calf Stretch ✌ | p. 101 | |

# Day 4

| | | |
|---|---|---|
| 1 The Monkey | p. 146 | |
| 2 Arm Circles: Free Standing | p. 105 | |
| 3 Standing on One Leg | p. 132 | |
| 4 Pelvic Stability Exercises – choose any two | p. 73 | |
| 5 The Starfish | p. 82 | |
| 6 Spine Curls | p. 91 | |
| 7 Hip Flexor Stretch | p. 94 | |
| 8 Side Rolls | p. 95 | |
| 9 Neck Rolls and Chin Tucks | p. 84 | |
| 10 Curl Ups | p. 120 | |
| 11 Oblique Curl Ups | p. 121 | |
| 12 Foot Exercises | p. 141 | |
| 13 Side Reach against the Wall | p. 106 | |
| 14 The Diamond Press | p. 136 | |
| 15 The Star | p. 115 | |
| 16 The Big Squeeze | p. 114 | |
| 17 The Rest Position | p. 118 | |

**Day 5**

|  |  | |
|---|---|---|
| 1 Windmill Arms | p. 99 | |
| 2 Spine Curls | p. 91 | |
| 3 Adductor Openings | p. 124 | |
| 4 Neck Rolls and Chin Tucks | p. 84 | |
| 5 Oblique Curl Ups | p. 121 | |
| 6 Dumb Waiter on the Wall | p. 108 | |
| 7 Floating Arms | p. 79 | |
| 8 The Oyster | p. 112 | |
| 9 Deep Gluteal Stretch against the Wall | p. 144 | |
| 10 The Dart | p. 138 | |
| 11 Table Top – whichever stage you are comfortable with | p. 134 | |
| 12 The Rest Position | p. 118 | |
| 13 Side Rolls | p. 95 | |
| 14 Hamstring Stretch | p. 122 | |
| 15 Foot Exercises | p. 141 | |
| 16 Arm Openings | p. 152 | |

**Day 6**

|  |  | |
|---|---|---|
| 1 Walking on the Spot plus Calf Stretch | p. 101 | |
| 2 Chicken Wings on the Wall | p. 126 | |
| 3 Standing or Sitting Waist Twists | p. 130 or p.131 | |
| 4 Spine Curls | p. 91 | |
| 5 Side Rolls | p. 95 | |
| 6 Neck Rolls and Chin Tucks | p. 84 | |
| 7 Curl Ups | p. 120 | |
| 8 Hamstring Stretch | p. 122 | |
| 9 The Oyster | p. 112 | |
| 10 Side-lying Quadriceps and Hip Flexor Stretch | p. 150 | |
| 11 The Diamond Press | p. 136 | |
| 12 The Big Squeeze | p. 114 | |
| 13 Knee Swings | p. 110 | |
| 14 The Cat | p. 148 | |
| 15 The Rest Position | p. 118 | |

# Day 7

| | | |
|---|---|---|
| 1 Pelvic Stability Exercises 👉 | p. 73 | |
| 2 Spine Curls 👌 | p. 91 | |
| 3 Hip Flexor Stretch 👌 | p. 94 | |
| 4 Neck Rolls and Chin Tucks 👉 | p. 84 | |
| 5 Oblique Curl Ups 👌 | p. 121 | |
| 6 Shoulder Drops 👉 | p. 86 | |
| 7 Side Reach against the Wall 👌 | p. 106 | |
| 8 Dumb Waiter on the Wall 👌 | p. 108 | |
| 9 The Diamond Press 👌 | p. 136 | |
| 10 The Star 👌 | p. 115 | |
| 11 The Cat 👌 | p. 148 | |
| 12 The Rest Position 👌 | p. 118 | |
| 13 Side Rolls 👌 | p. 95 | |
| 14 Hamstring Stretch 👌 | p. 122 | |
| 15 Adductor Openings 👌 | p. 124 | |
| 16 The Monkey 👌 | p. 146 | |
| 17 The Cushion Squeeze 👌 | p. 154 | |

# Daily Workouts for When You Are Feeling Fragile!

The following workouts avoid rotation and flexion (bending forward), and are ideal to do on days when you feel you need a gentler workout.

**Day 1**

| | | |
|---|---|---|
| 1 The Relaxation Position 👉 | p. 61 | |
| 2 The Compass 👉 | p. 62 | |
| 3 Lateral Breathing 👉 | p. 67 | |
| 4 The Pelvic Elevator 👉 | p. 68 | |
| 5 Pelvic Stability Exercises: Leg Slides and Knee Drops 👉 | p. 73 | |
| 6 The Starfish 👉 | p. 82 | |
| 7 The Dart: Stage One 👉 | p. 79 | |
| 8 The Rest Position 👉 | p. 118 | |
| 9 Neck Rolls and Chin Tucks 👉 | p. 84 | |

**Day 2**

| | | |
|---|---|---|
| 1 Alignment in Standing 🖢 | p. 66 | |
| 2 The Compass against the Wall 🖢 | p. 64 | |
| 3 Stabilizing on All Fours 🖢 | p. 70 | |
| 4 The Dart: Stage One 🖢 | p. 77 | |
| 5 The Rest Position 🖑 or the Relaxation Position 🖢 | p. 118 or p. 61 | |
| 6 Pelvic Stability Exercises: Leg Slides and Knee Folds 🖢 | p. 73 | |
| 7 The Starfish 🖢 | p. 82 | |
| 8 Hip Flexor Stretch 🖑 | p. 94 | |
| 9 The Cushion Squeeze 🖑 | p. 154 | |

**Day 3**

| | | |
|---|---|---|
| 1 The Relaxation Position 👆 | p. 61 | |
| 2 Pelvic Stability Exercises: Leg Slides and Knee Drops 👆 | p. 73 | |
| 3 Hip Flexor Stretch ✌ | p. 94 | |
| 4 Foot Exercises ✌ | p. 141 | |
| 5 The Big Squeeze ✌ | p. 114 | |
| 6 The Dart: Stage One 👆 | p. 77 | |
| 7 The Rest Position ✌ | p. 118 | |
| 8 Arm Circles: Free Standing ✌ | p. 105 | |
| 9 Standing on One Leg ✌ | p. 132 | |

**Day 4**

|  |  | |
|---|---|---|
| 1 The Compass against the Wall | p. 64 | |
| 2 Arm Circles: Free Standing | p. 105 | |
| 3 Dumb Waiter on the Wall | p. 108 | |
| 4 Walking on the Spot plus Calf Stretch | p. 101 | |
| 5 The Monkey | p. 146 | |
| 6 The Relaxation Position | p. 61 | |
| 7 Pelvic Stability Exercises: Knee Folds | p. 73 | |
| 8 The Dart: Stage One | p. 77 | |
| 9 The Cat | p. 148 | |
| 10 The Rest Position | p. 118 | |
| 11 The Cushion Squeeze | p. 154 | |

**Day 5**

| | | |
|---|---|---|
| 1 The Compass | p. 62 | |
| 2 Pelvic Stability Exercises: Leg Slides and Knee Drops | p. 73 | |
| 3 Hip Flexor Stretch | p. 94 | |
| 4 Shoulder Drops | p. 86 | |
| 5 The Starfish | p. 82 | |
| 6 Windmill Arms | p. 99 | |
| 7 The Dart: Stage One | p. 77 | |
| 8 The Rest Position | p. 118 | |
| 9 The Cushion Squeeze | p. 154 | |

## Day 6

| | | |
|---|---|---|
| 1 The Starfish | p. 82 | |
| 2 Hip Flexor Stretch | p. 94 | |
| 3 The Oyster | p. 112 | |
| 4 Stabilizing on All Fours | p. 70 | |
| 5 The Dart: Stage One | p. 77 | |
| 6 The Cat | p. 148 | |
| 7 The Rest Position | p. 118 | |
| 8 Knee Drops | p. 73 | |
| 9 Windmill Arms | p. 99 | |
| 10 Neck Rolls and Chin Tucks | p. 84 | |

**Day 7**

| | | |
|---|---|---|
| 1 The Starfish | p. 82 | |
| 2 Hip Flexor Stretch | p. 94 | |
| 3 The Oyster | p. 112 | |
| 4 Ankle Circles | p. 140 | |
| 5 Knee Drops | p. 73 | |
| 6 Dumb Waiter on the Wall | p. 108 | |
| 7 Arm Circles against the Wall | p. 103 | |
| 8 Standing on One Leg | p. 132 | |
| 9 Walking on the Spot plus Calf Stretch | p. 101 | |
| 10 The Cushion Squeeze | p. 154 | |

# The Full Back-Training Program

The following five workouts are for when you are strong enough to be able to include exercises from all three circles. If you have not yet reached Stage Three – the outer circle of exercises – you can always substitute another exercise from the inner circles.

## Workout 1

|  |  | |
|---|---|---|
| 1 The Starfish | p. 82 | |
| 2 Spine Curls | p. 91 | |
| 3 Hip Flexor Stretch | p. 94 | |
| 4 Hamstring Stretch | p. 122 | |
| 5 Pelvic Stability Exercises – choose any two | p. 73 | |
| 6 Neck Rolls and Chin Tucks | p. 84 | |
| 7 Oblique Curl Ups | p. 121 | |
| 8 The Dart | p. 138 | |
| 9 The Big Squeeze | p. 114 | |
| 10 Full Table Top | p. 168 | |
| 11 The Rest Position | p. 118 | |
| 12 Side Rolls or Hip Rolls | p. 95 or p. 164 | |
| 13 Single Leg Stretch | p. 178 | |
| 14 Windmill Arms | p. 99 | |
| 15 The Torpedo | p. 170 | |
| 16 The Oyster | p. 112 | |
| 17 Foot Exercises | p. 141 | |
| 18 Side Reach against the Wall | p. 106 | |
| 19 Chicken Wings on the Wall | p. 126 | |
| 20 Roll Downs | p. 161 | |

# Workout 2

| | | |
|---|---|---|
| 1 Walking on the Spot plus Calf Stretch | p. 101 | |
| 2 Arm Circles: Free Standing | p. 105 | |
| 3 Roll Downs | p. 161 | |
| 4 The Pelvic Bridge | p. 159 | |
| 5 Side Rolls or Hip Rolls | p. 95 or p. 164 | |
| 6 Neck Rolls and Chin Tucks | p. 84 | |
| 7 Adductor Openings | p. 124 | |
| 8 Single Leg Stretch | p. 178 | |
| 9 Windmill Arms | p. 99 | |
| 10 Ankle Circles | p. 140 | |
| 11 The Hundred | p. 182 | |
| 12 The Diamond Press | p. 136 | |
| 13 Butt Scrunches | p. 166 | |
| 14 Knee Swings | p. 110 | |
| 15 The Cat | p. 148 | |
| 16 The Rest Position | p. 118 | |
| 17 Abductor and Adductor Lifts | p. 174 or p.176 | |
| 18 Deep Gluteal Stretch against the Wall | p. 144 | |
| 19 The Cushion Squeeze | p. 154 | |

# Workout 3

| | | |
|---|---|---|
| 1 Shoulder Drops | p. 86 | |
| 2 Spine Curls with Cushion Squeeze | pp. 91, 154 | |
| 3 Neck Rolls and Chin Tucks | p. 84 | |
| 4 Curl Ups | p. 120 | |
| 5 Oblique Curl Ups | p. 121 | |
| 6 Knee Circles with Breath | p. 97 | |
| 7 Side Rolls or Hip Rolls | p. 95 or p.164 | |
| 8 Hamstring Stretch | p. 122 | |
| 9 Roll Downs | p. 161 | |
| 10 Chicken Wings on the Wall | p. 126 | |
| 11 Standing or Sitting Waist Twists | p. 131 or p.130 | |
| 12 The Hundred | p. 182 | |
| 13 The Diamond Press | p. 136 | |
| 14 The Cat | p. 148 | |
| 15 Butt Scrunches | p. 166 | |
| 16 The Rest Position | p. 118 | |
| 17 The Oyster | p. 112 | |
| 18 Side-lying Quadriceps and Hip Flexor Stretch | p. 150 | |
| 19 Deep Gluteal Stretch against the Wall | p. 144 | |
| 20 The Torpedo | p. 170 | |
| 21 The Cushion Squeeze | p. 154 | |

## Workout 4

|  |  | |
|---|---|---|
| 1 Walking on the Spot plus Calf Stretch | p. 101 | |
| 2 Standing on One Leg | p. 132 | |
| 3 Arm Circles Against the Wall | p. 103 | |
| 4 Dumb Waiter on the Wall | p. 108 | |
| 5 The Monkey | p. 146 | |
| 6 Standing or Sitting Waist Twists | p. 131 or p.130 | |
| 7 The Pelvic Bridge | p. 159 | |
| 8 Hip Flexor Stretch | p. 94 | |
| 9 Side Rolls or Hip Rolls | p. 95 or p.164 | |
| 10 Ankle Circles | p. 140 | |
| 11 Hamstring Stretch | p. 122 | |
| 12 Neck Rolls and Chin Tucks | p. 84 | |
| 13 Single Leg Stretch | p. 178 | |
| 14 The Dart: Stage Two | p. 138 | |
| 15 The Star | p. 115 | |
| 16 The Big Squeeze | p. 114 | |
| 17 Knee Swings | p. 110 | |
| 18 The Rest Position | p. 118 | |
| 19 Abductor and Adductor Lifts | pp. 174, 176 | |
| 20 Roll Downs | p. 161 | |
| 21 Arm Openings | p. 152 | |

# Workout 5

| | | |
|---|---|---|
| 1 The Starfish | p. 82 | |
| 2 Spine Curls | p. 91 | |
| 3 Adductor Openings | p. 124 | |
| 4 Side-lying Quadriceps and Hip Flexor Stretch | p. 150 | |
| 5 Backstroke Swimming | p. 177 | |
| 6 The Diamond Press | p. 136 | |
| 7 The Star | p. 115 | |
| 8 Table Top – whichever stage you are comfortable with | pp. 134, 168 | |
| 9 The Rest Position | p. 118 | |
| 10 Neck Rolls and Chin Tucks | p. 84 | |
| 11 Shoulder Drops | p. 86 | |
| 12 The Hundred | p. 182 | |
| 13 Standing or Sitting Waist Twists | p. 131 or p.130 | |
| 14 Side Reach against the Wall | p. 106 | |
| 15 Dumb Waiter on the Wall | p. 108 | |
| 16 One-legged Calf Raises | p. 172 | |
| 17 Roll Downs | p. 161 | |
| 18 Foot Exercises | p. 141 | |
| 19 Arm Openings | p. 152 | |
| 20 The Cushion Squeeze | p. 154 | |

# Lifestyle Tips for Living with Back Problems

In this section, we will be taking a look at some of the simple ways in which you can protect your back while carrying out daily activities. Hopefully, by following the Body Control Pilates Back-Training Program, your back will slowly become stronger, but it makes good sense to protect it as much as possible to help prevent further injury.

# Sitting

Ask yourself how many hours a day do you spend sitting down. Add it all up and you will be surprised at the amount! A Western lifestyle involves many sedentary activities including driving, eating, socializing, watching television, playing computer games, spending the day at office work-stations and commuting.

We believe that prolonged sitting is partly to blame for the huge increase in back-related problems. While sitting, the spine experiences twice the stress than it does when standing (see chart page 4). Worse still, a lot of the activities we do seated also involve leaning forward – for example, tying up shoe laces – which stress the spine even further.

The single most important thing to remember is to keep the natural "S-curve" of the spine (see page 8). Do not slouch.

Pointers for good sitting:

1  Sit on your sitting bones. You can feel these when you sit on a hard chair and place your hands under each buttock. By transferring your weight from cheek to cheek, you can feel the sitting bones. The weight should be evenly distributed between those bones. Try to keep your pelvis in neutral (see page 62).

2  Your feet should be planted firmly on the floor, hip-width apart.

3  Your thighs should be parallel or slightly sloping downward to the floor, the lower part of your legs at 90° to the thighs.

4  The height of the chair is very important: if it is too high your feet will dangle, in which case you should use a footstool or have your feet on a telephone book; if the seat is too low, a problem with some sofas, you increase the pressure on the lower back because it is much harder to maintain the natural curves of the spine. Chairs or sofas that are too soft, too low or too deep will not encourage you to sit well. Initially they might feel relaxing, but this is short lived.

5  Avoid crossing your legs because this twists your spine and restricts circulation in the legs.

6  Keep your back long with its natural "S curve" still present. When you are slouching you are making a "C curve" and are therefore increasing the pressure on joints and discs.

7  Supporting the lower (lumbar) back is sometimes necessary, especially if your core stabilizing muscles are not yet strong enough to do the job. A good chair provides this support, but a lumbar roll or a small cushion can be equally effective – and you can take them wherever you go!

8  Relax your shoulders and thighs.

9  Avoid sitting for long periods of time, especially if you are in pain. Move about every half an hour to stretch the back and decrease the pressure. Remind yourself to keep a strong center at all times.

10 The position of your head is very important. Your head is very heavy and can pull the spine out of alignment. Keep your neck soft and tension-free.

# Choosing a Chair for Sitting at Work

There are now many companies that specialize in ergonomically designed office chairs for back-pain sufferers.

Here are the most important things to look out for:

- Choose a chair where you can adjust the seat height and angle (see Sitting, Points 3 and 4 above).
- The ability to alter the angle of the seat during the day is very beneficial. A 5° angle is ideal. Posture wedges can also alter the angle of the seat.

- Back support is crucial and should also be adjustable to allow lumbar support.
- Armrests need to be exactly the right height, otherwise they can prevent you from sitting well. They should be low enough to go under the desk or you will be too far away from the workstation. They should support your arms, but not encourage you to lift your shoulders.
- Swivel chairs are beneficial because you can change position without twisting your back.

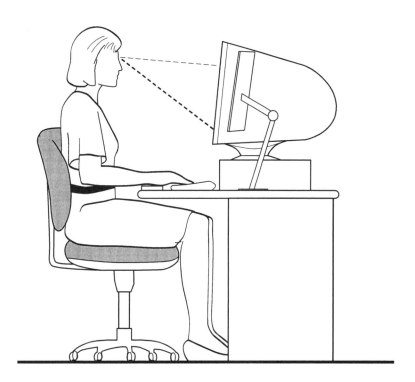

# At an Office or Workstation

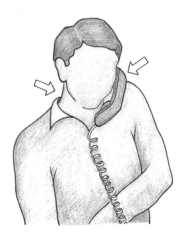 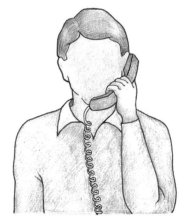

- The height of the desk is as important as the height of the chair. To determine the right height, bear in mind that when working on a computer, your forearms and wrists should be parallel to the desk top or sloping slightly downward from the desk.
- The height of any computer monitor is also crucial. You should not have to look down to see the screen as this causes tension in the neck and back. The center of the screen should be level with your eyes. Heighten the monitor if necessary.

- Your legs should be under the desk so that you do not have to reach forward to the keyboard. The desk should therefore be quite deep.
- Avoid cradling a telephone in your neck! Keep both shoulder blades down and your neck released. If you are a constant telephone user, use a headset or, if circumstances allow, a hands-free telephone.

# *Driving*

Driving may aggravate or cause back problems because it involves being in a fixed position for long periods of time, often in seats of poor design. Add to this the stress of driving in heavy traffic or with restless young children (or a mother-in-law) in the back seat, and it is not surprising that your back aches after a journey!

Here are a few tips to help you choose a back-friendly car:

1 Ask to test-drive a new car for at least an hour before you buy it to see if it is comfortable for you.

2 Make sure that the seat provides firm support beneath your butt and in the small of your back.

3 If possible, opt for seats that have an adjustable low-back support, both in terms of the size and the height of the support. This is a wonderful option because everyone's back is different and you can then alter the support to suit you.

4 If the seat does not have an adjustable lumbar support you may need to buy your own back support or posture wedge – or both.

5 Look to see if the pedals are central. They should not be positioned slightly off to one side or you will be driving in a twisted position.

6 Power steering and automatic transmission will help reduce the strain on your back.

7 The head restraint should not be so big that it alters your correct head and neck alignment.

8 If you know you will be lifting heavy luggage or other items into the trunk, then choose a car with a low trunk edge.

## When You Are Driving

- Remember all the good sitting directions on page 202.
- Try not to twist around awkwardly to get to the children (or the mother-in-law again) in the back seat. Stop the car and get out to deal with them.
- Take great care when lifting small children into and out of car seats. Try to avoid bending, twisting and lifting at the same time.
- Plan the journey to allow for plenty of breaks, and use this time to stretch your legs by walking around, rather than just sitting in the service station sipping coffee.
- If you are stuck in a traffic jam, you can practice your zip up and hollow and also do a few shoulder circles to release tension in the shoulders.

# Sleeping

A good night's rest is vital to a healthy body. During sleep, a lot of the body's repair work at cellular level takes place, allowing the body to regenerate itself. This applies especially to the injured body because damaged tissue needs time to heal. Many back-pain sufferers report restlessness in bed and sleepless nights. Problems sleeping will increase stress responses in the body and increase muscle spasm and, as a result, the pain cycle is perpetuated.

1 The choice of bed is important; it should be supportive and comfortable. If the mattress is too soft, your back will not be supported, and if it is too hard it does not "give" at your shoulders and hip and you will therefore lose the natural curves of your spine.

2 The bigger the bed the better. The more space you have to move around the less likely you are to sleep in one awkward position.

3 If you tend to sleep on your back, you might find a cushion under your knees helps to release the lower back.

4 Do not use too many pillows under your head, especially when you are sleeping on your stomach, since this will increase the arch in your lower back and strain your neck.

5 Prolonged sleeping on your stomach can strain your back; a cushion under your abdomen can alleviate this.

6 If you sleep on your side, make sure that you keep your spine aligned (see below). A cushion between your knees can make you more comfortable, especially if you suffer from sciatica.

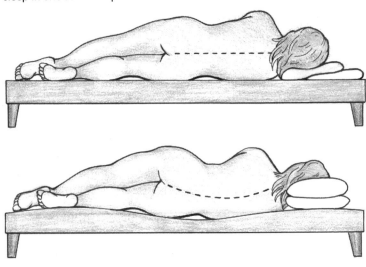

# Lifting and Carrying

One look at the chart on page 4 will tell you that lifting is potentially the most dangerous action for back-pain sufferers, especially if you combine it with twisting and bending. Good technique is very important in preventing back problems, but also allows your back to heal if it is already strained or damaged.

In an ideal world you should avoid lifting heavy loads completely if your back is fragile. If you cannot avoid lifting, at least take note of the following advice:

1 Where possible take the time to divide the load. It may take a little longer to complete the task, but it is better than harming your back.
2 Don't be afraid to ask someone to help you. An extra pair of hands will lighten the load.
3 When you are about to lift something, it is important to position yourself correctly to start with.

- You should be aware of the weight of the object that you are about to lift.
- Stand as close as possible to the load and have your feet on either side of it, with one foot slightly in front of the other, just as if you were going to take a step.
- Don't bend at the waist; bend at the knee and hip – the position is something like doing the Monkey exercise on page 146.
- Keep your back long and strongly supported by zipping up and hollowing.
- Keep your body close to the load, use handles, or place one hand under the object with the other hand on top. The further away you hold the load the more you are straining your back.
- Lean forward and, while maintaining a long back, straighten your knees and hips.
- Avoid lifting and twisting at the same time. Lift first and then rotate the whole trunk around to where you want to go.
- Avoid carrying a heavy load on one side of your body; try to divide it into equal weights.
- When lowering the load, reverse the above advice.

# Sex

If you suffer from back pain, it is going to affect every aspect of your life, including your sexual relationships. Hopefully, your partner will be sensitive to your problem but back problems are not immediately visible and sometimes it is very difficult for partners to be aware of your pain. Back problems can lead to sexual difficulties because the fear of pain can prevent you from enjoying sex; this may, in turn, cause frustration on both sides. Remember, a good sex life is important for a healthy body.

It is vital that you communicate any fears you may have to your partner. He or she needs to be aware of your concerns. That way, you can explore positions that enable you to continue to have sex and, more importantly, enjoy it. Generally speaking, you need to be comfortable and your partner has to "fit in." As far as possible, you should try to remain in an "S shape" position with the natural curves of your back maintained, which is the position of the woman's back in the illustrations. It is also important that you do not bear too much weight. We have given you several different positions to try in the diagrams below.

The most important thing is to give each other feedback, and to stop if it hurts. There are many ways of enjoying sex and, who knows, you might have lots of fun discovering new positions!

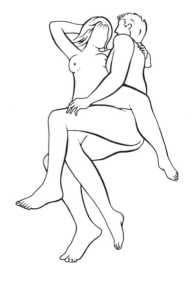

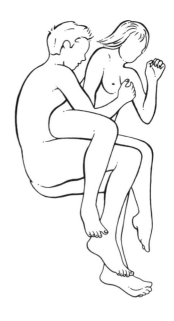

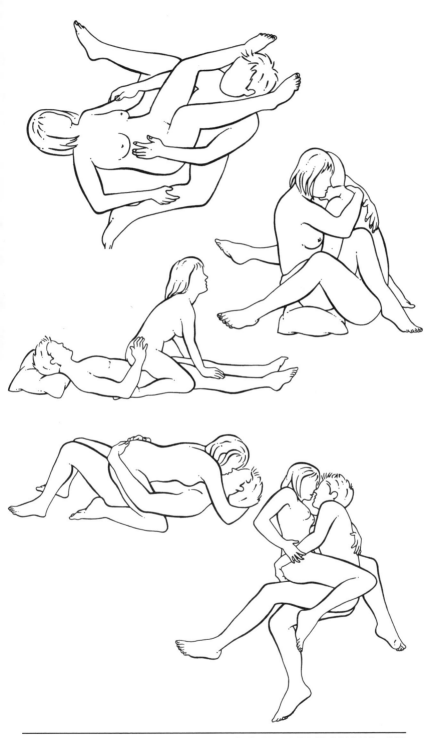

# Gardening

Gardening is an activity that is quite a challenge for back-pain sufferers. Over 400,000 people need medical attention every year after injuring themselves working in the garden. Our own clients often report increased pain and stiffness after a weekend's gardening.

Spring is the most common time for garden-related back problems. After a winter of inactivity there are a lot of strenuous jobs to be done in the garden, many involving heavy manual labor. We may remember to warm up the body before playing sport but few of us think about warming up before gardening, yet this is advisable. A few simple exercises, done both *before* and *after,* will help reduce injuries. Include some stretches in your preparation and wind down.

In particular be wary of weeding and planting since they involve gripping, twisting and pulling, which put great strain on your back. Stop frequently to stretch out the body, changing position and activity often. Most gardening tools now come with very long handles, which is helpful because they will prevent you from overreaching. Weeding is probably best done in a kneeling position as close as possible to the area being weeded.

If your back does not like extension (that is, bending backward), be particularly careful when pruning overhead branches. Do not overreach. When digging and shoveling, stand correctly (see page 66), let your knees take the strain rather than your back, and use a long-handled spade. While lifting, keep your back as straight as possible, remembering all the good lifting techniques on page 217. Wherever possible, divide the load and use a wheelbarrow to make several trips to the compost heap. If pulling up shrubs, crouch down as close as possible to the shrub, feet shoulder-width apart. Lengthen through the top of the head, bend your knees and slowly straighten the legs, zipping up and hollowing and keeping your back as straight as possible. Think of the Monkey on page 146. If you are sweeping leaves, hoeing or hedging, try to keep to a forward and backward action rather than an awkward twist. You should also vary the activities to use different positions and muscle groups.

Be kind to yourself when choosing a lawnmower, and choose a good-quality machine that is light and easy to use, rather than one that requires a lot of heavy pushing and pulling. If you chose a hover mower, try not to swing from the waist but turn your whole body in a line with the mower.

Above all, do not try to do everything in one day just because the sun is shining! It is better to do things in the garden little and often, rather than all at once.

# Commonly Asked Questions

**My doctor advised painkillers for my acute episodes of back pain. Is it advisable to take them?**
Yes, it is important to take analgesia at regular intervals. Start with acetaminophen, then substitute that with a non-steroid anti-inflammatory such as ibuprofen and then acetaminophen-weak opioid compounds. The type and frequency of the medication should be advised by your pharmacy or your general practitioner.

**I have gained a lot of weight after having my second baby. I am wondering if this is the cause of my back pain?**
The weight in itself is not the cause of your back pain, but the change in posture or the way you move may be the cause. By all means aim to lose some weight but also follow the guidelines as to when you should seek medical help (page 42). Then, when you are ready, you can start our back-training program.

**Whenever I go on vacation my backache seems to disappear. Could it be stress related?**
The discomfort may be related to the way you use your back on a daily basis. You need to take note of your posture while you work and undertake your other daily activities. Repetitive movements or sustained postures are probably the cause and, of course, these will be different on vacation.

**My doctor advised swimming to strengthen my back. Which stroke is preferable?**
Swimming is a good form of exercise to help strengthen your back because it uses large muscle groups. However, how you swim is crucial; you must choose an appropriate stroke or you will risk further damage to your back. The important considerations are the posture you maintain in the water and what things normally cause you back pain.

If bending forward is normally uncomfortable, then the breaststroke may be helpful – but you must ensure the position of your neck is correct so you don't pull on it too deeply, as well as not push your trunk too far into extension. If arching backward is uncomfortable, then backstroke may be helpful. Treading water is also a good way to strengthen muscles. Above all, there must be no increase in pain while you swim.

**Why does my backache seem worse in the mornings?**
A possible cause of this type of pain relates to the source of the pain in the joint and/or the disc. If the joint is held still for a period of time (while you sleep) and then you move, pain may result. Furthermore, the position in which you sleep may aggravate your symptoms. Follow the advice given on page 216. Remember, a healthy disc has the ability to absorb fluid when you sleep, i.e., when it is not acting as a shock absorber. If the disc is damaged, this ability is lost, hence the pain.

**When does backache become chronic?**
If you experience pain in your back for longer than four to six weeks from its onset, then the problem can be considered to have become chronic.

**What can a physiotherapist do for my backache?**
A physiotherapist will make a clinical assessment of the problem you are experiencing by asking you questions and undertaking specific tests and movements to help determine a more complete diagnosis. This enables them to give the correct treatment and to determine specific exercises for you to do. A better understanding of what and why the problem has come about will help in the eventual management of the problem.

**When should I stop exercising?**
If a specific exercise or an exercise regime causes or aggravates pain, then either you are doing the exercise incorrectly or it may not be suitable for you. None of the exercises in this back-treatment program should cause you discomfort either during or after they have been performed. If they do, you should stop immediately and get some expert advice. A medical practitioner can advise you as to whether a particular exercise is suitable or not. A qualified Body Control Pilates teacher will be able to check that you are doing the exercises correctly. You should also make sure that you are not pushing yourself too hard or trying to include too many new movements too soon. Slowly, gently and gradually build up your strength so that you exercise more safely and achieve more lasting longer-term results.

**I am thirty-four years old and my doctor has diagnosed degenerative changes in my neck. Is it unusual to have this at my age?**
All our joints undergo some change once we have passed the age of twenty-five, but the degree of change, or how it affects you, will be determined by the way you use your neck. Your condition may be due either to your posture or to a trauma (injury, accident) that you have experienced. But there are still things you can do to help. Go ahead with all the exercises gently and pay particular attention to the warnings we have given as to when the exercises are not suitable for anyone with neck problems – for example, Curl Ups would be contra-indicated and therefore not suitable.

# Glossary

**Acute** A problem that is less than forty-eight hours old.

**Analgesic** Describes the group of medications that help in the control of pain.

**Ankylosing Spondylitis** A chronic inflammatory disorder that affects the ligaments of the spine, relating to those influencing the spinal vertebrae. The ligaments become hardened due to the change in form, i.e., they become more bone-like or ossified. The pain is aggravated by excessive exercise and not completely relieved by rest. Symptoms include spinal stiffness and immobility, with the pain usually worse in the first hour of the morning. Gentle exercises such as those detailed in this training program are recommended and attention must be paid to good posture at all times.

**Anterior** In the front of your body.

**Cartilage** The covering of the joint surface that keeps the surface smooth in order to allow good movement.

**Cervical Spine** The top seven vertebrae of your spine to which your head is attached.

**Chronic** A long-standing condition, i.e., of more than forty-eight hours' duration.

**Concentric** A muscle contraction whereby the muscle shortens.

**Disc** Intervertebral discs between the vertebrae consisting of cartilage tissue that is 80 percent water. They are made up of two parts: the outer ring (annulus fibrosis) and the inner ring (nucleus pulposus). The discs act as shock absorbers (see page 3).

**Disc Bulging** The nucleus has moved but the annulus remains intact.

**Disc Prolapse** The disc has bulged, the annulus may or may not have torn depending on the extent of the bulge.

**Disc Rupture** The nucleus has moved, the annulus is torn and the disc extrudes. This is usually more serious than a disc bulge.

**Eccentric** A muscle contraction whereby the muscle lengthens while under tension.

**Epidural** Injection of an anaesthetic or other substance into the outside lining of the spinal canal.

**Extension** Bending the spine backward.

**Facet Joint** Paired joints that connect the back portion of the vertebrae (see page 5).

**Flexion** Bending the spine forward.

**Hypermobility** An increase in the relative range of movement of the joint.

**Hypomobility** A reduction in the relative range of movement of the joint.

**Isometric** A muscle contraction whereby, when the muscle is contracted and tense, there is no movement in the length of the muscle.

**Kyphosis** A description of posture whereby there is an increase in the thoracic curve and rounding of the shoulders. It is usually associated with the head poking forward (see page 20).

**Ligament** A band of fibrous tissue that connects the bones to the cartilage and supports and strengthens joints (see page 6).

**Lordosis** A forward curve in the lumbar spine caused by an excessive hollow in the lower back (see page 20).

**Lumbago** A description of pain in the lumbar spine, bruising in nature. A term rarely used today.

**Lumbar** The lower five segments of the spine.

**Osteoarthritis** A general term referring to degenerative changes to bone and cartilage caused by wear and tear of a joint (see page 10).

**Osteoporosis** A condition of the bone that leads to loss of bone density, resulting in a weakening of the bone (see page 10).

**Posterior** The area at the back of the body.

**Prolapsed Disc** see *Disc Prolapse*.

**Proprioception** The sense of balance and position of the limbs in space.

**Sacroiliac Joint** The joint between the sacrum and the pelvis. There are two sacroiliac joints, one on each side (see page 9).

**Scoliosis** An abnormal curve, or list, of the spine to the side. The degree of curvature can vary. Often not problematic (see page 8).

**Spondylosis** A degenerative change of the spine, which includes the vertebrae, the discs and the facet joints.

**Spinal Canal** The canal through which the spinal cord passes, formed by a tube through the vertebrae stacked on top of each other.

**Spinal Stenosis** An abnormal narrowing of the spinal canal.

**Synovial Fluid** Fluid produced by the lining of a joint (synovial membrane), which helps the joint to move smoothly.

**Tendon** A band of dense fibrous connective tissue that attaches a muscle to any part of the body.

**Thoracic Spine** The area in the middle of the back comprising twelve vertebrae.

**Vertebra** A bone of the spine. Each vertebra is made up of the vertebral body, the transverse process and the spinous process (see page 1).

**Whiplash Injury** A condition of the cervical spine, caused by a sudden change in movement of the spine in a forward or backward direction, resulting in potential damage to the soft tissue (ligaments and muscles) and sometimes the vertebrae. Leads to pain and restriction in the active movement of the spine.

# The Origins of Pilates and the Development of the Body Control Pilates® Method

## Joseph Pilates

Born in 1880 in Düsseldorf, Joseph Pilates was a frail, sickly child who suffered from rickets, asthma and rheumatic fever. Determined to overcome this fragility, instead of following an established fitness regime he experimented with many different approaches. Yoga, gymnastics, skiing, self-defense, dance, circus training and weight training all influenced him and he chose aspects of each to develop his own body. By absorbing these methods and selecting the most effective aspects, Joseph Pilates was able to work out a system that had the perfect balance of strength and flexibility.

Having proven his techniques on his own body, he then began to apply them to others. When World War I broke out he was training detectives at Scotland Yard but was classed as an alien and interned in Lancashire and later on the Isle of Man. With time on his hands, he helped out in the camp infirmary and further developed his techniques, training his fellow internees with amazing success. Many of his early trainees were war veterans with horrendous injuries such as amputations, and much of his knowledge of rehabilitation comes from this era.

At the end of the war he returned to Germany, where he taught self-defense to the Hamburg police and to soldiers in the German army. In 1926, he decided to emigrate to the United States. On the boat across he met his future wife Clara and, when they realized they shared the same views on fitness, they set up a studio together in New York, which soon attracted top ballet dancers (many sent from George Balanchine and Martha Graham), actors and actresses, gymnasts and athletes all anxious to learn from him.

Joseph Pilates wrote several books on fitness; the exercises described in these are very advanced and reflect the nature of his studio clientele. Pilates' interest was in the overall health of his clients. He advocated skin brushing long before it became generally popular and was also keen on the benefits of fresh air on the body – he would often teach *al fresco* in his swimming trunks! A major theme running throughout his work is that you must have commitment to the exercises; no excuses, they have to be done regularly in order to realize results.

Pilates never set up an official training program, with the result that many of his disciples went on to teach their own versions of his method. The definition of what was, or is, true Pilates is somewhat blurred and, indeed, is still being debated today. It is not helped by the fact that Joseph Pilates rarely taught the same exercise in the same way two days running because he geared his teaching to the needs of the individual and prescribed a completely different set of exercises for each client. Some of these clients themselves went on to teach, each one therefore working with a different emphasis.

Joseph Pilates died at the age of eighty-seven as a result of a fire in his studio.

# The Development of Body Control Pilates

Pilates has now been taught for some ninety years and yet it is only in the last few years that the medical profession has really begun to look closely at why the system is so successful. Because of this many Pilates teachers have taught intuitively, learning during apprenticeship about good alignment and good body use, but in many cases without fully knowing the medical rationale for what they are doing. Now under the close scrutiny of the medical world, we have had to re-examine our methods and study precisely why they work so well.

There is a common philosophy at the root of all Pilates-based methods that stems from the manner in which you approach the exercises – it is less about *what* you do, more about *how* you do it! This has been a great advantage to Pilates teachers because they have been able to absorb new ideas (for example, in physiotherapy techniques or movement therapies) and incorporate them into the method without sacrificing its uniqueness. As a result, Pilates continues to evolve as a system, to move forward without the constraint of a rigid set of rules.

The Body Control Pilates Method has evolved from the work of Joseph Pilates and been developed by Lynne Robinson, Helge Fisher and Gordon Thomson. Body Control Pilates is unique in the way it prepares the body for the classic exercises. Few people today could start their first session with the Hundred (page 182) as was traditionally the case. We believe that you need to acquire the skills to perform such exercises gradually. This progressive approach has won the respect and support of leading medical bodies as well as top sports associations.

# About the Authors

**Lynne Robinson** is a best-selling author who has co-written eight Pilates books. She is well-known for developing at-home, mat-based Pilates programs. Pilates expert **Helge Fisher** has co-authored *Pilates through the Day* and *Official Body Control Pilates Manual* with Lynne Robinson. **Paul Massey**, a physiotherapist, specializes in the prevention of sports injury. He is a qualified Body Control Pilates instructor and runs a Pilates studio in the U.K.

# References

Hodges, P. W., "Dysfunction of Transversus Abdominis Associated with Chronic Low Back Pain," *MPAA Conference Proceedings*, 1995.

Kendall, F. P., *Muscle Testing and Function,* Williams and Wilkins, 1993.

Keys, S., *Back Sufferers Bible*, Vermilion, 2000.

Maitland, G., *Vertebral Manipulation,* Butterworth, 1986.

Norris, C., "Spinal Stabilization," *Physiotherapy Journal*, vol. 81, no. 2, February 1995.

O'Sullivan, P. B., "Evaluation of Specific Stabilizing Exercises in the Treatment of Chronic Low Back Pain," *Spine*, 1997.

O'Sullivan, P. B., "Altered Abdominal Muscle Recruitment in Patients with Chronic Back Pain," *Journal of Orthopaedic and Sports Physical Therapy*, vol. 27 (2), 1998.

Panjabi, "The Stabilizing System of the Spine," *Journal of Spinal Disorders*, 1992.

Richardson, C. A. and Jull, G. A., "Pain Control. What Exercises Would You Prescribe?," *Manual Therapy*, vol. 1 (1), 1995.

# Further Information

For details about your nearest qualified teacher visit the Body Control Pilates website at www. bodycontrolpilates.com, where you can also find information on introductory workshops, Pilates vacations, home equipment and international Pilates contacts, or send a stamped addressed envelope to:

*The Body Control Pilates Association*
PO Box 29061
London WC2H 9DZ
England

For information on teacher training courses, please write to:

*Body Control Pilates Education Ltd*
14 Neal's Yard
London WC2H 9DP
England
e-mail: info@bodycontrol.co.uk
Tel: 44 (0)20 7379 3734
Fax: 44 (0)20 7379 7551

If you represent a sports or medical body and would like to receive details of specialist courses or programs run by the Body Control Pilates Group, if you are interested in introductory workshops, or if you would like to order Body Control Pilates books, videos, home or studio equipment please write to:

*Body Control Pilates Limited*
14 Neal's Yard
London WC2H 9DP
England

## General Information in the United States

*Balanced Body Inc.*
7500 14th Avenue, Suite 20
Sacramento, CA 95820-3539
Tel: 1-800-PILATES

Other overseas teachers can be found on the Body Control Pilates website at www.bodycontrolpilates.com

## Other Resources

The following organizations may also be useful:

*American Physical Therapy Association*
1111 North Fairfax Street
Alexandria, VA 22314-1488
www.apta.org

*American Osteopathic Association*
142 East Ontario Street
Chicago, IL 60611-3604
312-202-8000
800-621-1773
312-202-8200 fax
www.aoa-net.org

*American Academy of Physical Medicine and Rehabilitation*
One IBM Plaza, Suite 2500
Chicago, IL 60611-3604
312-464-9700
312-464-0227 fax
www.aapmr.org

*American Orthopaedic Society for Sports Medicine*
6300 North River Road, Suite 500
Rosemont, IL 60018
www.sportsmed.org

*www.spine-health.com*
Complete information on back health and pain, including referrals and tips

# Other Ulysses Press Books

**ELLIE HERMAN'S PILATES MATWORK PROPS WORKBOOK:**
**STEP-BY-STEP GUIDE WITH OVER 200 PHOTOS**
*Ellie Herman, $12.95*
Explains how props can enhance Pilates: the magic circles tone arms, the small ball held between the legs shapes thighs, the foam roller stretches the chest and shoulders, and the large exercise ball builds core stability.

**ELLIE HERMAN'S PILATES WORKBOOK ON THE BALL:**
**ILLUSTRATED STEP-BY-STEP GUIDE**
*Ellie Herman, $13.95*
Combines the powerful slimming and shaping effects of Pilates with the low-impact, high-intensity workout of the ball.

**THE JOSEPH H. PILATES METHOD AT HOME:**
**A BALANCE, SHAPE, STRENGTH & FITNESS PROGRAM**
*Eleanor McKenzie, $16.95*
This handbook describes and details Pilates, a mental and physical program that combines elements of yoga and classical dance.

**PILATES PERSONAL TRAINER BACK STRENGTHENING WORKOUT:**
**ILLUSTRATED STEP-BY-STEP MATWORK ROUTINE**
*Michael King and Yolande Green, $9.95*
The easy starter program in this workbook teaches Pilates exercises that are appropriate for strengthening the back in a safe and healthy manner.

**PILATES PERSONAL TRAINER GETTING STARTED WITH STRETCHING:**
**ILLUSTRATED STEP-BY-STEP MATWORK ROUTINE**
*Michael King and Yolande Green, $9.95*
Ideal for beginners or older people, the specially designed Pilates exercises in this book offer a gentle workout of light strength movements and key stretches.

**PILATES WORKBOOK:**
**ILLUSTRATED STEP-BY-STEP GUIDE TO MATWORK TECHNIQUES**
*Michael King, $12.95*
Illustrates the core matwork movements exactly as Joseph Pilates intended them to be performed; readers learn each movement by following the photographic sequences and explanatory captions.

*To order these books call 800-377-2542 or 510-601-8301, fax 510-601-8307, e-mail ulysses@ulyssespress.com, or write to Ulysses Press, P.O. Box 3440, Berkeley, CA 94703. All retail orders are shipped free of charge. California residents must include sales tax. Allow two to three weeks for delivery.*